SEIZURES, EPILEPSY, AND YOUR CHILD

SEIZURES, EPILEPSY,

A Handbook for Parents,

AND YOUR CHILD

Teachers, and Epileptics of All Ages

By JORGE C. LAGOS, M.D.

HARPER & ROW, PUBLISHERS

NEW YORK, EVANSTON
SAN FRANCISCO
LONDON

1817

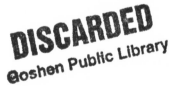

Grateful acknowledgment is hereby made for permission to reprint the material specified:

Excerpt from *Pediatrics*, Vol. 42. Reprinted by permission of the American Academy of Pediatrics.

Table on page 232 from article entitled "Childhood Epilepsy of Subcortical (Centrencephalic) Origin" by Julius D. Metrakos, Ph.D., and Katherine Metrakos, M.D., from *Clinical Pediatrics*, Vol. 5, September 1966. Reprinted by permission of *Clinical Pediatrics* and the authors.

Graphs on pages 84 and 85 from *Differential Diagnosis in Pediatric Neurology* by Jorge C. Lagos, M.D. Reprinted by permission of Little, Brown, and Company.

Excerpt from *Epilepsy and the Law* by Roscoe L. Barrow and Howard D. Fabing. Reprinted by permission of Harper & Row, Publishers, Inc.

Excerpts from Report of the American Medical Association Committee on Exercise and Physical Fitness from "Convulsive Disorders and Participation in Sports and Physical Education," *J.A.M.A.*, Vol. 206, November 4, 1968. Reprinted by permission of *J.A.M.A.*

FIRST EDITION

Designed by Sidney Feinberg

Library of Congress Cataloging in Publication Data
Lagos, Jorge C
  Seizures, epilepsy, and your child.
  1. Epilepsy in children. I. Title.
[DNLM: 1. Epilepsy—Popular works. WL385 L177e]
RJ496.E6L33   618.9′28′53   74–5792
ISBN 0–06–012504–7

To Heidi, Christine, and David

Contents

Preface

Approximately four million people in the United States have epilepsy, and several million other people who do not have epilepsy will experience, nevertheless, one or more seizures at some time in their lives.

Throughout history the epileptic has been considered to be possessed by supernatural influences or evil spirits, and his condition has been associated with mental retardation or insanity. Despite the fact that epilepsy is a common disorder, the epileptic is still today the subject of much bias and prejudice. It is not by chance alone that those who are physically handicapped—the blind, the deaf, the cerebral palsied—have enjoyed the sympathy and compassion of their fellow men. Man has always been able to close his eyes and realize what it is like to be blind, or place his hands over his ears and become aware of what it is like to be partially deaf. But no simulated experience can tell him what it is like to be epileptic. Little wonder that the epileptic, out of the ignorance of his peers and the unjustified fears bred by it, has been mercilessly stigmatized for such a long period of time.

And I am not referring to the Middle Ages. Until 1957, seventeen states prohibited epileptics from marrying, and nineteen states had provisions for the involuntary sterilization of epileptics. Until 1968 immigration laws prohibited epileptics from entering this country, even when they intended to come only for medical attention. Also until recently the epileptic was denied enrollment in many public schools, and in many states he was not allowed to drive a motor vehicle even if his seizures had been well controlled for many years. He was also refused life, health, and automobile insurance by most insurance companies, and was discriminated against by employers. The truth is that the epileptic was less than a second-class citizen, he was a second-class human being.

In the past forty years, medical science has gained a great deal of insight into the nature of epilepsy. It has also made remarkable progress in its diagnosis and treatment. The knowledge accumulated during this period of time has made untenable the many old wives' tales about epilepsy. In this age of enlightenment, there are no possible reasons left to justify biases and prejudices based entirely on ignorance.

During the past two decades the American public has become acquainted with some of the facts about epilepsy. This has been due, almost exclusively, to the unremitting efforts of a number of national as well as local organizations such as the Epilepsy Foundation of America, and to articles which have appeared in newspapers or popular magazines. To some extent these efforts have been successful. Officially, at least, the epileptic is no longer a second-class citizen. My conviction is, however, that at a "gut" level he is still one. I believe it is extremely difficult for people to get rid, in a short time, of prejudices which have for ages been passed on from one generation to another.

In spite of the great advances made in the field of epilepsy, the amount of information readily available to the general public is, to say the least, scanty. Worse yet, some of what is available, including short chapters in medical books for the layman written by physicians, is inaccurate, misleading, or obsolete. Because of the scarcity of material on seizures and epilepsy designed specifically for a general audience, I have felt the need to write this book, as one whose daily work deals in great part with children who have epilepsy or seizures.

My primary purpose has been to give parents of these children a clear and realistic view of their children's problems. With this in mind, I have sought to answer a number of queries that many of these parents have, and also to dismiss a number of their misconceptions. Adult epileptics should also find it useful, since they too may be the victims of inadequate or inaccurate information, as well as of prejudice and ostracism.

I do not pretend that parents of children with seizures or epilepsy have asked me all the questions I have formulated here. Far from that. Even the casual reader will see for himself that, because of the question-and-answer format I have used to make the subject easier to follow, a large number of the questions can only be the product of my own contriving. Nor is that all. I have also taken the liberty of putting in my own words those questions most parents do indeed ask.

It is my hope that this book will increase the public's understanding of what today is still one of the most misunderstood human conditions.

I am indebted to Sheryl Murtaugh for reading an early manuscript and making helpful suggestions, to Ann Harris, my editor at Harper & Row, for her invaluable editorial assistance, and to Robbie Kramer for her patience in the typing of the manuscript.

SEIZURES, EPILEPSY, AND YOUR CHILD

1. Epilepsy and Seizures

What is epilepsy?

The term epilepsy is derived from the Greek words *epilepsis* meaning "a seizure" and *epilambanein* meaning "to seize upon." There is ample historical evidence that epilepsy is an illness which has affected man since the dawn of history. Reference to this disorder has been found in Greek documents dating as far back as the twentieth century B.C.

Hippocrates (460-377 B.C.), a Greek physician, also called the Father of Medicine, wrote about 400 B.C. a monograph *On the Sacred Disease* (as convulsions were called in those times), in which he maintained that epilepsy was an illness that had its origin in the brain. Up to Hippocrates' time it was widely accepted that all diseases that affected man were the direct result of divine influences from a number of different gods upon a given individual. It is said that ancient Greek physicians were able to identify a particular god by the form that a seizure took. Hippocrates, on the contrary, believed that epilepsy as well as other diseases which afflicted man were not of divine origin but were due to abnormalities in the function of one or more organs of the human body. During the following two thousand years, Hippocrates' concept of the cause of epilepsy was completely dismissed by physicians and all sorts of other theories were postulated

1

instead. Some of these disparate theories included attributing seizures to sexual excesses or sexual aberrations, or to supernatural factors. For two thousand years, different versions of the Bible referred to individuals who were possessed by evil spirits during attacks which in retrospect appear to have been epileptic in nature. In line with present-day knowledge, the revised version of the New Testament (Matthew 17:15) states: "Lord, have mercy on my son, for he is an epileptic and suffers terribly, for often he falls into the fire and into the water."

Thomas Willis, an English physician of the seventeenth century, attempted to convince his contemporaries that seizures were brief, transient attacks which originated in the brain. Dr. Willis's effort apparently was not much more successful than Hippocrates'; the medical world of his time appears to have paid little attention to his revolutionary ideas.

The modern era of the study of epilepsy began in 1885. In that year Hughling Jackson, a British physician, postulated that epilepsy was a condition caused by "occasional, sudden, excessive, and disorderly discharges of nerve cells" in the gray matter of the brain. Gray matter is the name given to the parts of the brain where the body of nerve cells are found in groups of varying size. The remaining parts of the brain, called white matter, are made up of long, thin branches which arise from the bodies of nerve cells and whose role is to connect nerve cells from one to several other areas of the brain. The final proof that Hippocrates and Hughling Jackson's ideas were correct didn't come until half a century later when investigators began to study the electrical activity of different human organs and tissues. In 1929, Hans Berger, a German physician, invented the electroencephalograph (brain-wave-test machine), and with it he was able to demonstrate that a temporary disturbance in the electrical activity of the brain was the underlying cause of all epileptic seizures. He also showed that these transient abnormalities in cerebral function could be picked up by electrodes attached to a person's scalp and recorded permanently by pen writers on a running band of paper. In that year the electroencephalogram or brain-wave test was born, a diagnostic tool which would soon become the most important laboratory test in the study, diagnosis, and treatment of epilepsy.

All this information about the history of epilepsy sounds quite interesting, but so far you have not answered the first question. Or have you?

No, I have not. And the reason is easy to understand. It is not a simple task to define epilepsy. Webster's New World Dictionary of the American Language tells us that epilepsy is a chronic disease of the nervous system characterized by convulsions and often unconsciousness. And physicians, more than two thousand years after Hippocrates first suggested the same general concept, state that it is a chronic disorder of brain function characterized by seizures which are due to abnormal, sudden, transient, electrical discharges. The bad thing about these definitions is that neither of them is entirely satisfactory or comprehensive. The reason it is so difficult to give a more complete and all-encompassing definition of this disorder is that epilepsy is not a specific or a single chronic disease of the brain. *It is only a symptom, a manifestation of abnormal cerebral function which may be due to a large number of different causes.* Consequently, no matter what definition one comes up with, there will always be a number of patients who will not fit into it. As we will later see, the causes of epilepsy are not only many but they are also extremely varied. They can range from very small scars on the surface of the brain, not uncommonly the result of a mild birth injury, to extremely rare diseases of the brain in which an abnormality in one of the many chemical processes which are indispensable for the proper functioning of nerve cells is inherited from one or both parents.

How many people in the United States have some form of epileptic seizures?

Nobody knows for sure. Since epilepsy is not a contagious disorder, physicians do not have to report their patients to public health authorities. This is, however, only one factor which makes it difficult to obtain reliable figures with any degree of accuracy. An additional factor that complicates the gathering of reliable statistics is that some adult epileptics or some parents of epileptic children, because of the prejudices still surrounding epilepsy, conceal the existence of the disorder.

Most textbooks of medicine mention that one out of two hundred persons is affected with some sort of epileptic seizures. These estimates, largely based on figures collected at the time of military drafts, have been quoted repeatedly over the past fifty years without having been the subject of critical analysis. Thus far, comprehensive studies of the incidence of epilepsy in large segments of the population have not been conducted. Most medical authorities consider these figures as very conservative estimates. Physicians specializing in the diagnosis and treatment of people with epilepsy believe that the number of individuals suffering from some type of epileptic seizures is much higher, probably in the order of one per fifty persons in the general population.

Is the incidence of seizures the same in different parts of the world?

Yes. Seizures occur with equal frequency in all countries and all races. Males are affected as often as females.

Is the incidence of epileptic seizures the same in children as in adults?

No. Epileptic seizures occur much more frequently in children than in adults. It has been estimated that in approximately 80 percent of all cases of epilepsy, the first seizure occurs during the first two decades of life. Seizures occur most commonly at three periods in life: during the first two years, between four and eight years, and during adolescence. Owing to the increased risk of birth injury, the incidence of seizures is higher among first born. Nonepileptic seizures also occur more frequently in children than in adults.

Why are seizures more common in children than adults?

Several reasons can be given to explain this difference. First, the immaturity of the central nervous system in early life makes the brain much more vulnerable to just about any kind of injury. We should remember that despite an extremely long and complicated prenatal assembly line the infant-to-be develops from only two very small cells, the ovum from the mother and the sperm from the father. However difficult it may be to believe, these two cells possess all the know-how and have all the necessary genetic material to multiply and eventually develop into a healthy newborn with many billions of highly specialized cells. Somewhere along this extremely complicated assembly line, a number of things can go wrong. The placenta, the maternal organ attached to the wall of the womb from which the fetus gets the raw materials needed to survive and to grow, may not function properly. When this happens, the delivery to the fetus of these raw materials (oxygen, sugar, fats and proteins) will be insufficient to support its normal growth and development. Bacterial or viral infections of the mother during pregnancy may be passed on to the fetus across the placenta. Thus far physicians know of several infections of this type that can seriously interfere with the development of the embryo (product of conception up to three months of gestation) or the fetus (between three and nine months of gestation). By the end of the third month of pregnancy, when the embryo becomes a fetus, most of its organs are already fairly well formed. Hence, maternal infections after the third month of pregnancy are much less likely to produce congenital (present at birth) defects. But, during the first three months of pregnancy, when organs are rapidly passing from one to the next stage of development, the chances that severe congenital defects may occur as a result of such infections are relatively high. Not infrequently maternal infections can affect several organs of the embryo or the fetus. Thus, there is always the possibility that, in addition to abnormalities of the brain, congenital defects of the eyes, ears, heart, or other organs may also occur. Last but not least, during labor or delivery, as well as during the first few days of life, babies are exposed to a number of highly risky situations. That this period of life is indeed a dangerous one is well exemplified by the fact that today, despite the advances made by medicine in the past thirty years, more children still die during the first month of life than during all the remaining years of infancy and childhood.

Has there been a decrease in the incidence of epilepsy as a result of the advances which have taken place in medicine and related disciplines during the past thirty years?

No. It would seem only logical to believe that the great advances which have taken place in medicine and related fields during the past thirty years might in some way have effected a decrease in the incidence of epilepsy. Unhappily this has not been the case. Quite the contrary, medical progress has been directly responsible for an increase in the number of people suffering from epileptic seizures. For one thing, improved obstetric care and the facilities nowadays available for the management of seriously ill newborn infants have made possible the survival of many who once would have died from serious congenital cerebral defects or severe cerebral trauma sustained at the time of birth. Furthermore, the availability of highly sophisticated mechanical methods to assist failing breathing, as well as the development of a large number of potent antibiotics, have made possible the survival of premature babies weighing sometimes as little as one and one-half pounds, and also of a large number of newborn infants and young children with serious infections of the nervous system such as meningitis or encephalitis. Unfortunately, among the large number of survivors of many of these conditions there is still a significant percentage who are left with various degrees of brain damage that later in life may be the source of recurrent epileptic seizures.

A similar situation has occurred in children born with other types of birth defects. For example, a large number of children with congenital heart defects, who twenty years ago had little chance of survival beyond infancy or early childhood, can now be successfully treated surgically. Either before or at the time of heart surgery, some of these children may suffer from various kinds of cerebral complications which eventually may also be a cause of recurrent seizures.

In addition, the great technological advances made in other fields of medicine, such as neurosurgery, permit today the successful treatment of patients with brain abscesses, severe head injuries, and some types of brain tumors, all of whom would have died not too many years ago. Again a significant number of the survivors from any of these conditions can also develop recurrent epileptic seizures.

Also in the past twenty years the frequency of serious head injuries in children has increased considerably. As we will see in a later chapter some of these injuries are accidental, others are due to parental abuse.

All these factors have brought about a *real* increase in the incidence of epilepsy. On the other hand, an *apparent* increase in the number of people with epilepsy has also been observed during the past thirty years. Among the reasons that can be given to account for this apparent increase are better means of diagnosis, especially the widespread use of electroencephalography, and also the fact that nowadays, as a consequence of a more-understanding attitude by the general public toward the epileptic, fewer people conceal epilepsy or a member of the family affected with the disorder.

Is there any difference in meaning between the word "seizure" and the word "convulsion"?

No. The words "seizure" and "convulsion" are used interchangeably by physicians to describe short-lasting attacks that originate in the brain and may take a variety of forms. It should be made clear that their site of origin, the brain, permits physicians to differentiate true epileptic seizures from other attacks that may bear a close resemblance to them, such as syncope, or temporary episodes of loss of awareness or loss of consciousness due to impairment in the functioning of organs other than the brain.

Unless otherwise specified, throughout this book the words "seizure," "convulsion," "spell," "attack," and "epilepsy" will be used interchangeably. I must admit that I don't particularly like the term "epilepsy" and in my daily practice seldom use it. Instead I have made it a custom to label children with recurrent epileptic seizures as having a "chronic seizure disorder" and to state whether this is due to known or unknown causes. For example, if a child has had recurrent epileptic seizures as a result of a brain contusion suffered in early infancy, it is more appropriate to say that he has a chronic seizure disorder secondary to brain trauma than to say he suffers from epilepsy. By using this type of terminology one is able to describe in more or less accurate terms what is wrong with the child. If we simply say that he has epilepsy, we are giving a poor description of his problem, and also we are not separating him out from hundreds of other children who may have similar episodes due to entirely different causes.

I do not particularly care for the word "convulsion" either, but for a different reason from the layman. For most people the term "convulsion" has a mysterious and ominous significance. For me it does not. Rather I use the word "seizure" for the simple reason that it has a much broader meaning. As we will see later in this chapter, there are many children who do not actually "convulse" during a seizure. Nevertheless, there will be a few times when I will use the word "convulsion," almost always when referring to grand mal seizures during which an epileptic child actually does experience convulsive movements of his body.

Why do you also use the words "spell" and "attack"?

Only for convenience, and because they describe very aptly what actually happens to a child during some types of seizures. And since I take care of such a large number of children with chronic seizure disorders, the word "seizure" simply pops up so often in my daily conversation that I look for synonyms. I must say I don't use the word "fit," ever; this is simply because I don't like it.

What actually happens in the brain at the time of a seizure?

To give a clear although rather simplistic explanation of what takes place in the brain at the time of a seizure, we could say that under normal conditions the several billions of brain cells of a normal individual behave in a way which is comparable to a group of poorly trained soldiers firing their ammunition at different times and in multiple directions. This lack of synchronized cerebral activity results in a large number of electrical discharges that balance one another out. When, for one of many possible reasons, a certain group of brain cells behaves in a highly synchronized manner, as would a well-trained battalion, all their electrical ammunition is fired simultaneously and in the same direction. The external manifestation of this synchronized and temporary outburst of electrical discharges may be a *seizure* or *convulsion*. It is not difficult to realize, then, that if a brief disturbance of the electrical activity of the brain is the direct cause of seizures, there can be nothing mysterious or magic about such seizures; they are simply the result of transient disturbances in the function of a group of brain cells. Actually, something similar happens when other organs of the human body do not function properly. There exists, however, a fundamental difference between the abnormalities in cerebral function which may cause epilepsy and the abnormalities in function due to diseases affecting other organs. When an organ other than the brain is diseased, symptoms are expected to occur more or less constantly. In contrast to this, and despite the fact that in most cases the brain abnormalities responsible for epilepsy are always present (a scar, for instance, is permanent), seizures occur only at variable intervals, sometimes several times a day, sometimes once a week, once a month, or only once a year.

The analogy between the well-trained battalion of soldiers firing their ammunition in a well-synchronized manner and the synchronized electrical brain discharges producing a seizure is not very convincing. If a well-trained battalion is the right type of battalion, what's wrong with a well-synchronized brain?

I have to admit that the analogy is, at best, a poor one. Although I tried very hard, I just couldn't come up with a better one. It was not until I had spent a few hours searching for the appropriate analogy that I realized I was actually wasting my time, for the simple reason that the normal state of affairs in a normal brain happens to be one of constant desynchronization, if not total chaos! For a number of reasons which I will not discuss here, what is good for a battalion or a kindergarten class is simply not good for the brain.

I would like to emphasize at this point the basic concept that the capacity to convulse is an intrinsic quality of the human brain. In this respect no human being is exempted. Given the right circumstances, anyone can have a convulsion. Thus, a person suffering from delirium tremens, or someone exposed to an electric current of high voltage, or an infant with severe dehydration due to vomiting or diarrhea may develop severe convulsions although none of them has ever had them in the past and never again in the future will have another one.

What do you mean when you say that the ability to convulse is an "intrinsic quality" of the brain?

Nothing more and nothing less than that. An intrinsic quality of a diseased liver, for example, is to produce jaundice; an intrinsic quality of the bowels is to produce diarrhea; and an intrinsic quality of human hair is either to fall out with aging or to become gray. If the right conditions are present, the human brain is always ready to cause a convulsion.

In order to get a clearer picture of what a seizure really is, we should remember that the primary, though not exclusive, role of the brain is to receive information from our environment, to process this information, and then to send back messages or directions about how to carry out in a smooth and coordinated manner every one of our daily activities from the time we wake up until we fall asleep. Not that during sleep the brain stops working. As we shall see in a later chapter, sleep is far from being a state of temporary death. But at least while we are asleep contact with our environment is minimal. To be able to perform even the simplest purposeful task it is necessary that we be constantly aware of what's taking place around us. To accomplish the simplest movement we need to be able to move in a coordinated manner several out of the more than two hundred different muscles of our body. We also have to be able to receive sensory information through our eyes, ears, skin, nose, tongue, and sense of balance at all times. Since these are basically the matters with which the nervous system is concerned, transient disturbances in the functioning of one or several areas of the brain may bring on a temporary breakdown in this normal relationship with our environment, the result of which may be a seizure or convulsion. Because seizures may arise from several areas of the brain, each of which is concerned with entirely different functions, epilepsy may manifest itself, as we will explain later, in many different forms other than the well-known attack characterized by sudden loss of consciousness and convulsive movements of the entire body.

Do epileptic seizures have something in common?

Yes, irrespective of the form they may take, all epileptic seizures share three main characteristics: their onset is always sudden, their duration varies usually from seconds to one minute or several minutes, and their ending is in most cases also abrupt. If a child has recurrent episodes that meet these characteristics and *whose place of origin is the brain,* we can say he suffers from epilepsy. It should be emphasized, however, that when we use the word "epilepsy" we are really not saying anything more about the *cause* of a child's recurrent attacks than if we say he has short-lasting, recurrent episodes of stomach ache, vomiting, or headache. If the precise cause of the seizure is known, it would probably be more appropriate to say that a child suffers from an "X" condition, of which the seizures may be its only manifestation, or that he suffers from a well-known disease of the brain, of which the seizures may be one of several symptoms or manifestations.

How many types of seizures or convulsions are there?

Quite a few. If we wish to compare seizures with anthropology, and come up this time with a better analogy, we could say that there are two races of epilepsy and in each race there are several nationalities. All varieties of epilepsy can be divided into two basic categories: primary and secondary. Primary epilepsy, also called essential or idiopathic (of unknown cause), is that in which the exact cause of the seizures cannot be determined with the diagnostic methods presently available. Secondary epilepsy, also referred to as symptomatic or acquired, is that in which the cause of the seizures, even if not precisely known, can at least be suspected on the basis of the child's past medical history, his physical examination, or the data provided by laboratory tests such as blood or urine tests, skull x-rays, or the electroencephalogram. To understand the difference between these two basic forms of epilepsy more easily, let's compare seizures with sweating and assume for a moment that two persons go to see a physician because of excessive sweating. After a complete examination the physician concludes that in one of the patients the cause of excessive perspiration is poor functioning of a heart valve. In this case the physician may say that this person suffers from excessive sweating which is *secondary* to an identifiable and more or less well-known cause. On the other hand, an equally extensive medical investigation of the second patient sheds no light as to the cause of his excessive sweating. Nevertheless, even if the physician is unable to identify the cause of the problem, it is obvious that there must be something wrong with the sweat glands of the patient; for some unknown reason they just seem to produce too much sweat. The physician, however, is not satisfied with this simple but totally unsatisfactory answer, and refers the patient to a dermatologist who decides to remove a piece of skin (biopsy) in order to examine the abnormal sweat glands under the microscope. To his great surprise the dermatologist finds that the sweat glands look exactly like those found in people who perspire normally. The shape, the size, the internal structure, all the things of which a sweat gland is made up, appear to be entirely normal. The dermatologist can reach but one frustrating conclusion; although the many small building blocks which make up the sweat glands of the patient look completely normal there must be something in them that is responsible for the excessive sweating. Now in his ignorance he uses another term and says that the *function* or that the *metabolism* of the sweat glands is abnormal. For some reason which the microscope cannot reveal they are producing too much sweat.

What does sweating have to do with primary or secondary epilepsy?

Not much; but a situation comparable to the latter example exists in patients who are said to have *primary epilepsy.* Even if we were able to look at those groups of live brain cells from where seizures arise and watch them closely during the course of an attack, we would be unable to tell that they actually looked any different from those of another individual who has never had seizures. In a way we can say that a group of brain cells is sweating too much; that they are performing their function in an abnormal fashion; that something is wrong with their function or metabolism. Of course everybody knows that brain cells are not made to sweat. Brain cells, also called neurons, are highly specialized, very excitable cells which perform their functions by generating, receiving, and sending electrochemical messages from one part of the brain to another, and from the brain and spinal cord to just about everywhere else in the human body. When a seizure occurs in a patient with primary epilepsy, a group of brain cells, for a brief period of time, behaves in an abnormal way and give rise to a large number of highly synchronized electrical discharges. To put it in other words, for a brief period of time a group of these deceptively normal-looking brain cells stops doing its own thing and does something completely out of the ordinary.

Why and how does this happen?

Nobody knows for sure. The exact reason that seizures may occur in the absence of an obvious structural brain lesion remains unknown. Yet it is generally accepted that transient alterations in brain metabolism lower the seizure threshold (brain resistance to seizures) of deep midline brain structures which are concerned with the preservation of consciousness and posture. There can be little doubt that eventually the precise reason for this temporary lowering of brain resistance to seizures in individuals with primary epilepsy will be found to be a brief disturbance in one or more chemical processes within a group of cerebral cells. In the past few years, scientists have been able to maintain alive in culture media pieces of brain tissue from patients with epilepsy who have undergone surgery for the removal of an epileptogenic focus. Thus far they have found out that marked differences exist in some chemical reactions going on inside these epileptic nerve cells when compared with those of normal brain cells.

On the other hand, patients who are said to suffer from secondary epilepsy have a defect in the architecture of the brain which usually can be directly or indirectly demonstrated in one way or another. This lesion can be a small scar on the surface of the brain, which may be the result of birth trauma, or the aftermath of bacterial or viral infections (meningitis, encephalitis) of the brain or of its covering membranes, or may have been due to a large number of other causes.

The main causes of epilepsy will be discussed in Chapter 2.

The above-mentioned division of epilepsy into primary and secondary is of great importance not only because of their entirely different underlying causes, but also, as we will later see, because of the different implications from the standpoint of treatment, prognosis, and inheritance.

You have already mentioned several times that epileptic seizures may take several different forms. How many forms are there and how do they differ from one another?

From a purely descriptive point of view—that is, considering only what happens to a patient during an epileptic attack—there is more than one type of seizure. With this in mind we could divide seizures into two major categories depending on whether during an attack the child does or does not lose consciousness for any significant period of time. During a grand mal seizure the child loses consciousness and almost always experiences convulsive movements of the entire body. In the course of all other forms, on the other hand, the child either loses contact with his environment for periods varying from a few seconds to a few minutes or loses consciousness for only a very brief period of time, which seldom lasts longer than two or three seconds.

What are grand mal seizures?

For many years the word "seizure" and especially the word "convulsion" have been associated in the mind of the overwhelming majority of people with what is called "grand mal convulsion." *Grand mal* are French words that literally mean "great ailment." One could refer then to this form of epilepsy as a severe seizure or as a major convulsion. Grand mal seizures, the most common type (approximately 70 percent of all cases of epilepsy), doubtless the most dramatic, but fortunately also one of the easiest to prevent with appropriate treatment, are characterized by sudden loss of consciousness and sudden loss of muscle tone. Owing to these two factors, the victim falls immediately to the ground. This is almost always followed by stiffening of the entire body, clenching of the teeth, rolling of the eyes in various directions, foaming at the mouth, spasm of the larynx (tightening of the voice box), and sometimes loss of bladder or rectal control with involuntary urination or defecation. During the brief period of stiffening of the body and as a result of spasm of the larynx, the patient may stop breathing for a short period of time and his skin may acquire a bluish discoloration (cyanosis), especially around the lips, as a consequence of a temporary lack of oxygen. The period of stiffening (also called tonic phase), which lasts only a few seconds, is frequently followed by a second period, during which there is jerking of the four extremities (also called clonic phase), which, as a rule, lasts anywhere from one to twenty minutes. When this second phase is over, the child usually becomes limp and more often than not falls into a deep sleep (postictal state), which may last from a few minutes to several hours. If a grand mal attack is of short duration, the child may feel groggy for a few minutes afterward and then be back to normal as if nothing had happened. Occasionally during a grand mal attack a child may experience no jerking of his body. He may suddenly lose consciousness, fall to the ground, and then remain limp for one or more minutes.

What else can happen during or after a grand mal attack?

Not a great deal. Even though for the onlooker the sight of a person having a grand mal seizure may be an impressive experience, actually very little more than what has been previously mentioned happens to the child during the course of a major seizure or after the attack is over. As a matter of fact, and for reasons which we do not fully understand, victims rarely suffer bodily injury of any significance

as a result of the initial fall or as a consequence of the convulsive movements of the head, body, or extremities. For a
few hours following an attack the child may complain of sore
muscles. Serious injuries, however, occur only in very ex-
ceptional instances.

Also in rare cases, while the patient is still limp and in a
deep sleep (postictal state), a new seizure, which is similar,
more severe, or longer than the previous one, may develop.
Occasionally, this can go on and on for several hours, and
sometimes for one or two days. When grand mal seizures recur
at such short intervals we say that the child is in *status epilepticus*. These two words literally mean "epileptic state."
During this state, grand mal seizures recur in such rapid succession and at such brief intervals that the child passes from
one postictal stage to the other without regaining consciousness.

What can be done if a child should develop status epilepticus?

Only one thing, stop it. And, since there is nothing parents or well-motivated neighbors can do to accomplish this,
the child in status epilepticus should be taken to a hospital
as soon as possible. Grand mal convulsions taking place within
such a short span may sometimes completely exhaust the
brain or may seriously compromise its oxygen supply. Status
epilepticus is therefore a *true medical emergency*. It is always
possible that as a result of very frequent and prolonged grand
mal seizures the child may die of sheer cerebral exhaustion,
or that he may recover but be left with irreversible brain
damage. Either of these two possibilities is, however, an uncommon occurrence. More often than not, neither fatal nor
permanent damage occurs and the child recovers from the
prolonged episode without any signs or symptoms of brain
damage. From the preceding comments, then, it goes without
saying that status epilepticus should always be considered

a dangerous situation. Therefore, it is imperative that the child be taken as soon as possible to a hospital where he can receive prompt and appropriate treatment to stop the seizures and at the same time be given supportive care (oxygen, respiratory aid, intravenous fluids, etc.). At the present time physicians have at their disposal several excellent drugs for the treatment of this medical emergency. The sooner treatment is begun in a child in status epilepticus the better the chances of rapidly controlling seizures. Because of the great importance of the time factor, it is recommended that parents of children who have had more than one grand mal seizure within a short period of time or parents of children who have previously had an episode of status epilepticus have available at home a supply of anticonvulsant drug which can be administered by rectum.

Johnny's seizures don't seem to be of the grand mal type. Suddenly he may start jerking or having a few muscle twitches on one side of the body or in one arm or one leg. He doesn't seem to lose consciousness and doesn't fall. What type seizures does he have?

True, Johnny is not having grand mal seizures. In this case we are dealing with another type of seizure, which manifests itself as a sudden onset of muscle jerks in one part of a limb, an entire arm or leg or both, or at one corner of the mouth. This muscle jerking is not accompanied by loss of consciousness and seldom lasts longer than a few seconds, one or two minutes. Sometimes instead of having muscle jerking the child may experience a strange feeling (numbness, tingling) on one side of his body. Occasionally this type of seizure may progress in severity and develop into a grand mal seizure with loss of consciousness, stiffening of the body and jerking of the four extremities. This type of convulsion in which only one part of the body is involved and which

associated with impairment of consciousness is called a "focal seizure." This means that the abnormal electrical discharges causing the seizure can be traced to one small area (or focus) in the brain which is concerned with motion or sensation in that part of the body affected by the abnormal movement or feeling. If these focal seizures (jerking or abnormal feeling) occur on the left side of the body, the abnormal electrical discharges come from the right side of the brain and vice versa. This is simply because movement as well as feeling on the left side of the body is controlled by the right side of the brain and that of the right side of the body by the left side of the brain.

Some children may have, over a period of years, a number of *focal motor* (jerking) or *focal sensory* (abnormal feeling) seizures that are never followed by a grand mal seizure. In other children, however, a focal seizure may or may not, at different times, develop into a grand mal convulsion.

Why does this happen?

In patients with focal seizures (motor or sensory), the abnormal electrical brain discharges originate and remain localized during the entire spell within a small portion of the brain which controls body movements or receives sensory information from the environment. If the surrounding brain areas are not able to hold back the electrical discharges, they may spread to central areas of the brain which are concerned with the maintenance of consciousness and muscle tone and from the center of the brain to its entire surface. When this occurs a grand mal attack will develop.

Johnny, our three-year-old child, had his first grand mal seizure at the age of seven months at a time when he had an ear infection and a temperature of one hundred and four degrees. Since then he has had two other similar episodes and

on both occasions his temperature has also been very high. Otherwise he is a perfectly normal child. Does he have epilepsy?

Probably not. It is little known by the general public that a large number of young children, usually between the ages of six months and two years, may have convulsions in association with febrile illnesses (illnesses accompanied by high fever) such as a viral infection, an ear infection, a strep throat, or some of the other common illnesses of childhood. These so-called *febrile seizures* are always of the major type (grand mal), with loss of consciousness, stiffening of the body, and jerking of the four limbs. Since febrile seizures represent such a major problem in the practice of pediatrics, the magnitude of the problem should be immediately emphasized. It has been estimated that approximately 2 to 4 percent of all children under the age of five years will have, at one time or another, at least one or more febrile seizures. Usually the precipitating illness is an upper-respiratory infection, tonsillitis, or ear infection. Febrile seizures do not occur often during the course of the common childhood diseases such as measles, German measles or chicken pox, with the exception of roseola. Males are more frequently affected than females and white children more often than black children. The exact mechanism by which sudden elevations in body temperature due to the common illnesses of childhood can produce a grand mal convulsion in some children remains unexplained. For some reason, however, fever appears to lower the seizure threshold in only some of them and as a consequence of this phenomenon a brief, temporary, and self-limited outburst of cerebral electrical discharges takes place. Even though the precise mechanism that brings on febrile seizures is unknown, there can be little doubt that age and incomplete cerebral maturation play important roles. In most children febrile seizures do not last more than one to three minutes and rarely last more than twenty minutes. Seldom does a child have more than one seizure during the course of a single febrile illness. Febrile seizures occur most frequently early in the course of a febrile illness, usually two to six hours after the onset of fever. Rarely, if ever, will a febrile seizure occur in a child who has already had fever for more than twenty-four hours.

Febrile seizures do not necessarily occur each time a given child develops high fever. The average child who suffers from febrile seizures may have anywhere from two to five attacks. A small percentage of them will have only one attack and another small group will have more than five. Febrile seizures rarely occur for the first time before the age of six months or after the age of three years. And if a child has had febrile seizures early in life, they rarely recur after the age of five years.

Febrile seizures have a tendency to run in families. It has been estimated that in approximately 30 to 50 percent of cases, other family members have also experienced the same type of attacks during early childhood.

The prognosis for children who have had febrile seizures is excellent. In approximately 80 to 90 percent of cases these children will never again have seizures in association with febrile illnesses after the age of five or six years. The remaining 10 to 20 percent will eventually develop seizures in the absence of fever. With the exception of the children from the latter group there is no reason whatever to label as epileptics the thousands of infants or young children who have had one or more grand mal seizures only during febrile illnesses. (See page 95 for discussion of current concepts in the treatment of febrile seizures.)

If a child suffers from other types of recurrent attacks that also have their origin in the brain and during which he may

or may not lose consciousness, can he also be considered to have epilepsy?

Probably yes. It is surprising to what extent people have succeeded in their efforts to associate the words "epilepsy," "seizures," and "convulsions" only with one of the previously described forms of attacks. In all probability this misconception arose from the erroneous assumption that if a child does not convulse or shake violently during one of these episodes, he probably does not have epileptic seizures. Pediatric allergists often mention that "not everything that wheezes is asthma." We can paraphrase this sentence and say that *not all shaking spells are epilepsy and many nonshaking spells are.* In addition to the well-known grand mal attack, there are many other types of epileptic spells. And the fact that all of them are less dramatic than what we have already described doesn't make them less epileptic.

Let's re-emphasize at this point that when we talk about epileptic seizures we are referring only to those attacks which originate in the brain, as opposed to other types of episodes such as fainting spells, syncope, breath-holding spells, or other short-lasting attacks during which a person may experience transient loss of consciousness as a result of conditions in which there is a temporary decrease in the amount of blood reaching the brain. In a later chapter I will discuss the main conditions which can be confused with epilepsy.

Is it difficult to recognize these other types of epileptic seizures?

Sometimes. Some of the less well-known forms of epilepsy can manifest themselves as more or less inconspicuous episodes of such brief duration that they may go unrecognized for weeks and occasionally for months. This is really not difficult to understand if one considers that brief episodes of abnormal behavior, short-lasting spells of apparent daydreaming, or sudden, unexplained and inconsequential falls, all of them incidents that are not uncommon in childhood, may all be the result of recurrent seizure activity.

What are the names given to these "inconspicuous" epileptic seizures and how can one recognize them?

We mentioned earlier that the most common type of seizure, and the only one that many people associate with epilepsy is that in which there is sudden loss of consciousness along with shaking or convulsive movements of the body. These so-called grand mal seizures probably account for about 70 percent of all forms of epilepsy. The other types have been given the following names: petit mal, psychomotor, myoclonic, akinetic, and convulsive equivalents.

What do these complicated names mean? Why do physicians have to give such technical names to what is just another form of epileptic attack?

It shouldn't be difficult to understand that in order to differentiate one type of seizure from another physicians have had no choice but to give each of them a different name. The only purpose of these names is to describe, in each case, what a child does or what happens to him during an attack. One should remember that the ability to give a seizure its proper name is much more than just an academic or semantic exercise on the part of physicians. Since different types of seizures may require entirely different types of medication, it is obvious that the success in their treatment will depend almost exclusively on the ability of the physician to name correctly the type of seizure a child is having.

Because what happens to a child during a seizure is nothing to be taken lightly, and also because I am not going to take the risk of creating a credibility gap, from here till the end of this chapter, and off and on in subsequent ones, I will ask you to bear with me through passages of pretty dry, almost technical prose.

What are petit mal seizures?

Petit mal are French words which mean "small ailment," and, in a less literal although more fitting translation, "small attack," or "small seizure." Petit mal attacks are very short-lasting and inconspicuous seizures. They are, however, extremely stereotyped, almost always manifesting themselves in exactly the same way in a given child. Actually, petit mal attacks are such a stereotyped form of seizure that the episodes differ very little, if at all, from one child to another. Petit mal seizures are characterized by sudden loss of awareness, by a vacant and glassy stare, and by sudden interruption of the activity in which the child was engaged, including speech. During the spell, which lasts from four to thirty seconds, the child does not fall, nor does he lose upright posture or balance. There is no stiffening of the body or jerking of the limbs. Occasionally during an attack the child may make subtle swallowing movements or may smack his lips. In a matter of seconds the seizure is over and the child resumes whatever activity he was engaged in before the attack, and has no memory of having had one. A child with this type of seizure may have anywhere from a few to fifty or one hundred or more spells every day.

Petit mal attacks almost always have their onset between four and eight years of age, rarely recur beyond puberty, and almost never occur for the first time after the age of twenty years. Petit mal attacks rarely start prior to the age of four and probably never before the age of three years. Because of their very brief duration and the lack of associated muscle jerks, not infrequently the true nature of the attacks is first recognized by the child's teacher, who notices that his pupil is having what appear to be very frequent, short-lasting epi-

sodes of daydreaming. In some large families with several
siblings of school age, it is not at all uncommon for a child
to have had petit mal seizures for several weeks before his
parents become aware that the frequent lapses of awareness,
or the apparent short episodes of inattention or daydreaming,
are not really what they seem to be.

What are psychomotor seizures?

The term "psychomotor" is a combination of the words
"psyche" (mind) and "motor" (movement or motion). As its
name implies, then, during a psychomotor seizure there is a
combination of unusual mental behavior and inappropriate
motor activity. Psychomotor seizures are really not associated
with true loss of consciousness—or, at least, not with what
most people think of when they use the word "unconsciousness." During an episode the child does not fall to the ground
unconscious and does not remain totally unresponsive to his
environment. Instead, in the course of a psychomotor seizure,
the child suddenly loses contact with his environment and behaves as if he were totally unaware of what is going on around
him. This abrupt change from normal to more or less erratic
behavior may be accompanied by various automatic activities
and bizarre motor acts. The child may stop doing whatever
he was doing prior to the attack; he may have a vacant stare
or look around as if he suddenly found himself transported
to an entirely unknown and unexpected place; and not infrequently he may display a vague or frightened facial ex-
pression. While temporarily unaware that he is living in a
different world, he may smack his lips automatically, perform
meaningless swallowing and chewing movements, or purposeless and repetitive motions with his hands, such as tapping his
thighs or picking at his clothes, or he may just wander aim-
lessly about the room. Sometimes he may perform apparently
meaningful but irrelevant acts in relation to a given situation.

Here is an example: A ten-year-old boy had received a guitar for his last birthday. One morning at school, while class was in progress, he got up from his desk and walked to the back of the classroom. He acted as if he had opened a window where there was none and said in a loud voice to someone present in his imaginary world, "Bring me my guitar." As soon as he had said this, he went back to his seat, sat down, and resumed his classroom activities where he had left off.

Although psychomotor seizures may manifest themselves in any of the forms previously mentioned, all of them have in common a brief period of irrational or bizarre behavior that may last from a few seconds to several minutes. More often than not, psychomotor seizures are followed by a period of drowsiness or confusion.

What are myoclonic seizures?

The word "myoclonic" is made up of two words, *myo* (muscle), and *clonic* (jerks). Literally, then, it means a "muscle jerk." In this type of seizure, however, more than just one single muscle of the body is involved in the jerk. Myoclonic seizures may manifest in one of three main ways: (1) by a sudden forward flexion (nodding) of the head; (2) by a sudden flexion of the head and an upward jerking motion of the arms; or (3) by a sudden flexion jerk of the entire body (head, arms, and legs). If the muscle jerk is severe, the child may fall to the ground violently as if somebody had thrown him down. The seizure lasts only a few seconds, being over just about by the time the child hits the floor. If consciousness is lost, it is only momentarily. The child recovers immediately and, if he was standing and has fallen to the ground, gets up in a matter of seconds. Myoclonic seizures are not followed by drowsiness or sleepiness. As often happens in children with petit mal, myoclonic seizures also tend to occur several times daily. It is not uncommon to see a child who may have experienced frequent and unexplained falls for periods of weeks or months before his parents realize that the falls are not the result of accidental tripping, nervousness, or clumsiness.

What are akinetic seizures?

The word "akinetic" literally means lack of movement or motion and also lack of muscle tone. The term "akinetic" is used to describe a type of epileptic seizure which is characterized by sudden and very brief loss of muscle tone (which maintains a person in the erect position) and also very brief loss of consciousness. As a consequence of this the child suddenly goes limp and falls to the ground. He gets up from the floor in a matter of two to three seconds and immediately afterward feels fine and acts as if nothing had happened. Akinetic seizures also have the tendency to occur many times daily.

So that in grand mal, myoclonic, and akinetic seizures there is loss of consciousness of variable duration, and in petit mal and psychomotor seizures there is loss of awareness and loss of contact with the environment. Right?

Right.

What's the difference between "unconsciousness," "unawareness," and "loss of contact" with the environment?

Although I think I know exactly what the difference is, it is not easy to put it into a few words. Unfortunately, Webster's New World Dictionary of the American Language lists the word "consciousness" as a synonym of "awareness" and vice versa. To complicate things even further, the word "unconsciousness" is not equated with the loss of consciousness that occurs, for example, during a grand mal seizure or as a result of a severe blow to the head. According to accepted usage, when a prize fighter is knocked out, he is unconscious as well as unaware. When a person is under the influence of psychedelic drugs he may be unaware but he is not unconscious.

The definer of these words in the dictionary was probably not *aware* that a person can be totally unaware of what is happening to him while he is still conscious. During a grand mal seizure, the child, like the prize fighter, is unaware and unconscious; during a petit mal he is unaware of his surroundings but is still able to maintain his normal posture and to perform subtle and meaningless motions with his arms, mouth, and eyes; and during a psychomotor attack he may go around performing purposeless acts of which he is totally unaware while he's still obviously not in a state of unconsciousness. The problem is really a matter of semantics. The English language simply lacks a word to describe the state of a person who, for a brief period of time, is totally unaware of reality but is still, in more than one way, conscious. Temporary insanity, of course, won't do.

What are convulsive equivalents?

"Convulsive equivalent" is a term used to describe episodes characterized by the sudden onset of headache; paroxysmal abdominal pain, with or without nausea or vomiting; and bizarre nightmares or unexplained episodes of night or day terrors, caused by brief abnormal electrical discharges in certain areas of the brain. The most common form of convulsive equivalent is characterized by paroxysmal, episodic, and short-lasting episodes of abdominal pain. During the spell, which lasts not more than a few minutes, the child usually also shows some evidence of disturbed awareness or responsiveness to his environment. The attacks, as is the rule with all other types of seizures, begin and end abruptly. It is generally accepted that the temporary electrical brain discharges responsible for the recurrent episodes of headache or abdominal pain probably originate in deep midline cerebral structures which are concerned with a variety of body functions, such as the control of heart rate and blood pressure, which are not under the influence of our conscious mind. It should be admitted that a diagnosis of convulsive equivalent is not an easy one to make. Before a child is labeled as having repeated bouts of abdominal pain, vomiting, headache, or night terrors on the basis of abnormal electrical brain discharges, other much more common causes have to be ruled out by appropriate studies. The child may have a duodenal ulcer or some other intestinal problem, he may have migraine headaches, or he may be an emotionally disturbed child in need of psychiatric help rather than an antiepileptic drug.

After reviewing the many different forms an epileptic attack may take we can easily appreciate that, in addition to the well-known *grand mal* seizure, there are several other types of attacks which are also epileptic in nature and are also due to short-lasting and self-limited disturbances in the electrical activity of the brain.

What causes a child to have one type of seizure and another one to have a different type?

In order to answer this question we will need to repeat a few things which we have already discussed in previous pages. Depending on what happens to a child during an epileptic attack, the different types of seizures fall into several distinct forms. During an attack the child may lose consciousness, fall to the ground, and then exhibit stiffness of his body followed by jerking of the four limbs. He may have only muscle jerking or experience an abnormal feeling on one side of his body without losing consciousness. He may suddenly lose contact with his environment, performing automatic movements and behaving in a bizarre and meaningless way. He may have a sudden and rather violent jerk of his head, arms, and legs, fall to the floor, and recover almost immediately. He may suddenly become limp, fall to the ground, and then recover completely in a matter of one to two seconds. Or finally, he may experience recurrent episodes of abdominal pain, with or without vomiting, or headaches of sudden onset and sudden termination. All these forms in which a seizure may manifest itself have one thing in common: they are the result of a temporary outburst of abnormal cerebral electrical discharges.

The area of the brain from which those discharges arise determines whether one or another type of seizure will occur.

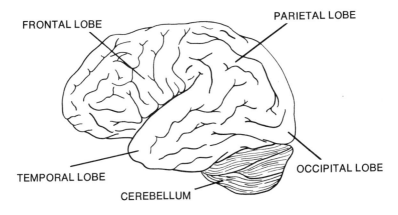

FRONTAL LOBE

PARIETAL LOBE

TEMPORAL LOBE

CEREBELLUM

OCCIPITAL LOBE

Fig. 1. Lateral view of brain showing its main lobes. Secondary grand mal seizures may arise from frontal, parietal, temporal, or occipital lobes. Focal motor seizures arise from frontal lobe, and focal sensory seizures from parietal lobe. Psychomotor seizures originate in temporal lobes. All other forms of seizures (primary grand mal, petit mal, myoclonic, akinetic, and convulsive equivalents) originate from deep midline brain structures. A focal motor seizure may become a secondary grand mal seizure when the electrical discharges spread from the surface of the brain to midline structures. Convulsive equivalents can also originate from temporal lobes and structures adjacent to them.

If the area of the brain where the seizure originates is a small portion of the surface of the brain that controls movements or body sensations, the result may be muscle jerking or an abnormal feeling limited to only one part of the body without associated loss of consciousness. If during the entire duration of the episode the discharges remain localized to that small part of the brain, nothing else will occur; if the discharges spread to other areas of the brain surface or to deep midline structures, a major convulsion (grand mal) will develop. The great majority of grand mal seizures which occur during the first four years of life originate in one small portion of the surface of the brain. They arise from a very discrete area, or focus, and from there they spread to the rest of the brain.

Psychomotor seizures which are characterized by brief periods of purposeless behavior almost always originate in one or both temporal lobes. The temporal lobes of the brain, which are located directly under the skull at about the level of the ears, have to do with a large number of body functions and, to a great extent, they determine also a person's behavior, personality, and memory. It is not surprising then that abnormal electrical discharges arising from one or both temporal lobes may cause loss of awareness and strange or bizarre behavior.

All other forms of seizures appear to be the result of electrical disturbances coming from central portions of the brain. Among many other functions, these areas are concerned with the maintenance of muscle tone (posture), alertness, awakening, sleep, and also the maintenance of awareness and consciousness. When a temporary impairment in the function of some of these structures takes place, the result may be sudden loss of awareness without loss of posture (petit mal); or abrupt and short-lasting episodes of loss of consciousness and loss of muscle tone (akinetic); or a sudden jerk of a part or the entire body accompanied by a very short loss of consciousness (myoclonic).

Central regions of the brain are also concerned with a number of body functions which are not under the influence of voluntary control (blood circulation, blood pressure, temperature, hunger, thirst, production of hormones, etc.). Thus, transient electrical disturbances in these areas may produce so-called convulsive equivalent attacks which are characterized by recurrent episodes of abdominal pain, headache, flushing, pallor, etc.

Do patients with epilepsy have some kind of a warning before an attack?

Yes. A number of patients experience some sort of warning or *aura* shortly before a seizure. The nature of the warning depends on the part of the brain from where the seizure arises. The most common type of warning is a strange feeling or sensation rapidly ascending from the stomach to the head. Other less-common warnings consist of ringing in the ears, dizziness, visual hallucinations, tingling in one corner of the mouth or in one extremity, smell hallucinations usually of a very unpleasant nature, or at times an undescribable feeling or fear that something very unusual is going to happen. If the site of origin of the seizure is a portion of the area of the brain that controls motion, the warning may consist of a slight involuntary movement or jerking of a finger, usually the thumb, or a muscle twitching in one corner of the mouth or in one side of the face. Older children soon learn that any of these warnings may be followed either by abrupt loss of consciousness or by more widespread and severe muscle jerking. Thus many of them are able to stop whatever they are doing at the time and get to a safe place.

Can a child have more than one type of seizure?

Yes. If one takes at random one hundred children with seizures, approximately 60 percent of them will have one type of attack, and the remaining 40 percent will have two or more types. Thus, it is not at all uncommon to see children who experience, at different times, more than one type of seizure. About 50 percent of children with petit mal, for example, have had or will eventually experience one or more grand mal seizures. The reverse, however, is not true. The number of children who suffer from grand mal and who also have other types of seizures is relatively small. Children who have minor motor seizures (myoclonic and akinetic) often also suffer from major motor attacks. Rarely a child may have as many as three different types.

2. What Can Cause Epileptic and Nonepileptic Seizures?

Why does Johnny have seizures?

This question is usually preceded or followed by one or more of the following sentences: "My husband and I are completely normal and as far as we can tell there has never been any member on either side of our family affected with convulsions, mental retardation, or anything else that has to do with the brain. As a matter of fact, Johnny is developing in all respects even a bit faster than our two older children. What causes Johnny's seizures? If something is found to account for the seizures, is there something that can be done about it? Does he have brain damage? And, if he has a normal brain, will seizures produce any brain damage? What will happen to him when he grows up to be a man? Will he be able to go to a regular school? Will he be able to get married and have children?"

These are only some of the most common questions that parents of children with seizures ask their pediatricians or their family physicians. From the outset I have to make clear that physicians are seldom able to answer that question which, although not the most important, is nevertheless from the parents' point of view the most puzzling and intriguing: "Why does Johnny have seizures?"

Why is that?

We have mentioned earlier that seizures are the external manifestation of sudden, abnormal electrical discharges in a certain region of the brain. Isn't this in any way an appropriate answer to the question? Of course it isn't. It cannot possibly leave a parent satisfied, for the simple reason that it is not a useful explanation. Indeed, such an answer is not only unsatisfactory, it is, as far as parents are concerned, downright meaningless. What the parents of a child with epilepsy want to know is what is *causing* the abnormal electrical discharges in their child's brain. And the truth is that at the present time, scientists and researchers throughout the world are also seeking a precise answer to the same question. Unfortunately, in our present stage of medical knowledge, physicians are unable to answer this fundamental question most of the time. Much more frequently than they would like, they have no alternative other than to give parents incomplete and sometimes vague answers. They base these answers on what is often an unreliable and nebulous medical history of the child, on the type of seizure the child has, on certain abnormalities which may be present in the electroencephalogram, and, occasionally, on the information provided by other laboratory tests such as skull x-rays, or blood or urine tests.

We have mentioned previously that seizures or convulsions are not a single disorder, but a symptom or manifestation of transient abnormalities in cerebral function which may be due to a variety of conditions affecting the brain. Seizures, although not epileptic in nature, can also be caused by the abnormal functioning of other organs of the body. For example, diseases of the pancreas or diseases of the parathyroid glands may intermittently lower the amount of glucose (sugar) or calcium in the blood. When the amount of these compounds in the blood falls below a critical level, a seizure may occur. Lowering of the blood levels of magnesium or vitamin B_6 can also produce seizures which are indistinguishable from seizures originating in the brain. Seizures due to a low blood level of magnesium or vitamin B_6 are extremely rare and occur almost exclusively in very young infants.

During the middle fifties an epidemic of seizures occurred in the United States in babies who were receiving a commercial milk substitute totally lacking in vitamin B_6. Since then no new cases have been reported. Also, in extremely rare instances, a baby is born with a congenital defect called vitamin B_6 (pyridoxine) dependency. As its name implies, babies born with this defect are "dependent" on vitamin B_6. For unknown reasons, infants so affected require a daily intake of this vitamin which is several times higher than normal. In babies born with vitamin B_6 dependency, seizures occur shortly after birth and cannot be controlled with any of the anticonvulsant drugs available at present. All convulsive activity ceases, however, within a few minutes after the intravenous or intramuscular administration of the vitamin. Vitamin B_6 dependency is a rare congenital metabolic defect and should not be construed as an argument to support the erroneous belief that "lack of vitamins" is a cause of seizures in older children. Convulsions due to a low blood concentration of any of the previously mentioned compounds (glucose, calcium, magnesium, and vitamin B_6), are always of the grand mal type.

By definition, a child who has seizures due to diseases of an organ other than the brain does not suffer from epilepsy but from conditions which under certain circumstances may produce seizures which are indistinguishable from those seen in children with epilepsy. Unfortunately, the number of children in whom recurrent seizures are due to remediable conditions such as a low blood concentration of any of the previously mentioned compounds is extremely small. In the great majority of children with a chronic seizure disorder, seizures are due to transient abnormalities in the metabolism of an otherwise normal brain, or are due to some sort of structural brain abnormality causing intermittent disturbances in brain function.

Structural brain abnormality?

Yes, I realize the term needs explanation. At best, "structural brain abnormality" is a good euphemism for what many people call brain damage. What brain damage really is, and more important, what the layman implies when he uses these two words, still escapes me. First of all let me confess, without shame, that I don't know what the brain of a normal person looks like, and I seriously doubt that anybody does. Moreover, I am fully convinced that nobody has such a thing as an entirely "normal" brain. What I am really trying to say in a rather circuitous way is that I believe all of us suffer from varying degrees of brain damage. If the reader believes that I'm blowing the issue out of all proportions, all he has to do is to think for just one moment of the two million people in the United States who have hearing loss of handicapping magnitude; or the six million who have some sort of speech or language problem; or the millions of individuals who, despite an average basic intelligence are incapable of learning to read well; and the millions who are totally unable to carry a tune, or are so overtly clumsy that they could never learn to play baseball or tennis. It doesn't really matter what euphemism one wishes to use to describe the reason for these people's difficulties; brain damage is as valid as any. It is about time to accept the fact that there is something "wrong" with the brains of many millions of human beings—much more than many of us realize or are willing to accept.

But what does all this have to do with the structural abnormalities that may be present in the brains of children with
epilepsy?

Quite a bit. In many children with epilepsy, what physicians call "structural brain abnormality" and people call
"brain damage" may be of no greater magnitude than the abnormalities in the brain of a person who doesn't hear well, or
of an individual who is so clumsy that he is incapable of
handling a hammer without crushing his fingers. In case you
want a bit of more-tangible proof, we can mention that in
many children who have had seizures for a number of years,
not even the most sophisticated laboratory test or the most
refined microscopic examination of small pieces of brain
tissue removed at surgery, or of the entire brain at autopsy,
provides clues regarding the precise nature of the abnormality that caused the seizures.

Until about thirty years ago and only because of limited
medical knowledge, primary or idiopathic epilepsy was the
most common type of epilepsy. Until recently everything
physicians didn't know they called "of unknown cause" or
idiopathic. With newer and better methods of diagnosis, the
number of cases falling into this category has decreased considerably. At any rate, there are still a certain number of
children with seizures, probably around 50 percent, in whom
the defect appears to be a metabolic abnormality of the brain
which causes periodic highly synchronized electrical discharges which may become externally manifested as seizures.
The remaining 50 percent of children with seizures are said
to have secondary or acquired epilepsy, in which an architec-
tural—that is, structural—abnormality in one or more areas
of the brain is present. These small areas of defective cerebral
architecture (usually scars) may be due to a number of different causes, such as birth trauma, severe head trauma during

early infancy or childhood, infections of the brain (encephalitis) or its covering membranes (meningitis), intoxications (lead poisoning, etc.) and a number of other much rarer causes such as brain tumors.

How important is birth trauma as a cause of seizures?

One of the most important. Birth trauma ranks very high among the main causes of seizures, and it can first manifest itself not only in the newborn period but also in infancy, in childhood, and even later on in life. In this respect it should be pointed out that not even the most normal pregnancy, labor, or delivery is a written guarantee that a newborn infant could not have suffered some minor injury in a small area of his brain which later in life, and not infrequently as late as thirty or forty years afterward, may become the triggering point (epileptogenic focus) of abnormal cerebral electrical discharges.

What can go wrong at the time of birth that may eventually lead to epilepsy?

A number of things. It is an old cliché that man takes too many things for granted. Birth is certainly one of them. We tend to forget that being born was probably one of the most traumatic experiences many of us will ever experience in life. It is well known that the pressure which the baby's head withstands throughout the process of delivery is, indeed, formidable. Fortunately, at birth, the bones of the skull are not yet fused and therefore can easily overlap in response to pressures from the outside. In addition to this, at birth the brain is smaller in relation to the inside of the skull than at any other time in extrauterine (outside the womb) life. These two factors are of great importance in the ability of the head of the fetus to withstand not only the great pressures but also the sudden changes which take place during labor and delivery. Just to give an example of how traumatic an experience birth can be, I should mention that in approximately 15 percent of newborn infants there is some bleeding between the surface of the brain and its covering membranes (meninges) and that in about 25 to 40 percent of newborns, small hemorrhages occur in the inner surface of the eyeballs, so-called retinal hemorrhages. In the overwhelming majority of births, however, these types of hemorrhages appear to be of no consequence.

We should hasten to add that not even babies born by Caesarean section are exempt from problems like these. To be sure, Caesarean section is by no means equivalent to an easy birth. In many instances this method of delivery is used after rupture of the bag of water (amniotic sac) when spontaneous vaginal delivery has already proved impossible. Frequently a Caesarean section is done because of serious maternal complications, and even if surgery is performed before rupture of the bag of water and the onset of labor, the head of the fetus is often very strongly pressed against the mother's hip bones before the beginning of labor.

In spite of all these possible complications, it is nonetheless surprising that the great majority of newborn babies are capable of going through this traumatic ordeal suffering little, if any, permanent brain damage.

Since during birth the head of the baby is subjected to such strong pressures from the outside that small bleedings may occur inside the eyes and on the surface of the brain, there is no reason to believe that the same thing does not sometimes occur inside the brain. It does. Of course, under different circumstances these hemorrhages can vary considerably in size and number. In most so-called normal deliveries, a number of very small hemorrhages probably occur inside the brain but are of no further consequence. In other cases the bleeding may arise from fairly large blood vessels and be of such magnitude as to represent an immediate threat to the baby's life. Between these two extremes there are infants who shortly after birth are in no danger and appear to be entirely normal, but in whom the bleeding may have been of such magnitude and have occurred in such a location as to become a source of problems later in life in the form of seizures, learning difficulties, or mild to moderate mental retardation.

If all this weren't enough, at the time of birth the brain may also suffer a concussion or a contusion (bruise) which is in no way different from that seen following serious injuries to the head later on in life. Both concussion and contusion of the brain at the time of birth may produce swelling and destruction of brain tissue in a manner which is similar to that observed in other parts of the body after severe trauma. Unlike other body tissues, however, brain tissue does not regenerate after destruction. To complicate things further, along with bleeding and swelling there may also be a decrease in the amount of oxygen reaching the brain of the baby, resulting in death of thousands of nerve cells in one or more relatively small parts of the brain. The only reason we say "relatively small" is that, although all of us can get along quite well with a bruised arm, nose, or liver, none of us can afford to lose even a very small piece of our brain.

In a fairly large number of babies, and even though some of the previously mentioned complications have taken place at the time of birth, the infant may still show no abnormal signs or symptoms of any kind during the early months of life. It may not be until several months or years after birth that symptoms related to birth injury, such as convulsions, may become apparent.

How common are seizures in newborn infants and what can cause them?

The incidence of seizures in the newborn period (first month of life), or in the neonatal period (first week of life) has been estimated to be anywhere between one in one hundred and fifty to one in five hundred live births. Most seizures in newborns occur during the first or second day of life. A large percentage of seizures during this period of life occur in prematures, in babies born of mothers who have had complicated pregnancies (toxemia, etc.), or in babies born after prolonged labor, difficult deliveries, or both. In many infants, however, seizures are due not to birth injury but to a temporary fall below a critical level in the blood concentration of certain substances such as glucose, calcium, or magnesium. Other causes of seizures in this period of life are congenital malformations of the brain, infections of the membranes covering the brain (meningitis) or infections of the brain proper (encephalitis), a transient decrease in the amount of oxygen reaching the brain (hypoxia) during labor or delivery, or bleeding inside the brain or over its surface due to severe trauma to the baby's head during delivery.

Seizures in newborns may also occur in babies whose mothers are drug addicts. Severe seizures and other symptoms in newborns of mothers who are drug addicts was a medical curiosity until about 1950. In the past twenty years this problem has become less unusual. Until the mid-1950's morphine was the usual addicting narcotic; since then the great majority of maternal addicts use heroin. Shortly after birth these babies experience what has been called the "narcotic withdrawal syndrome," which is characterized by extreme irritability, tremors, a high-pitched cry, nausea, vomiting, diarrhea, yawning, sneezing, high fever, and grand mal convulsions sometimes followed by shock and death. The mortality rate in babies with the "narcotic withdrawal syndrome" is extremely high if the condition is not recognized and treated in time. Convulsions can also occur in newborn babies of alcoholic mothers.

The correction of low levels of blood glucose, calcium, or

magnesium will stop seizures attributable to these causes. The outlook for newborn infants with meningitis is not as good as that in older infants affected with this disease. Mortality rate is still high, even with early and adequate treatment, and the number of infants left with some sort of cerebral injury is also high. The treatment of seizures and other manifestations seen in babies born of mothers who are drug addicts consists of the administration of a combination of paregoric elixir (tincture of opium) and Chlorpromazine (a tranquilizer) for two to six weeks. In other words, the baby is treated as if he were a temporary drug addict.

In about one-third of newborn babies a diagnosis as to the exact cause of seizures cannot be made. There can be little doubt, however, that in the great majority of these cases in which a diagnosis is not made, some kind of minor cerebral insult due to trauma during the process of delivery is responsible for the seizures.

Is there a way to predict how babies who have had seizures during the first few days of life will eventually develop?

Yes. The electroencephalogram has been found to be an important prognostic aid in determining how babies who have had one or more seizures during the first few days of life will eventually do in terms of mental and motor development. In one study of a large number of babies who had had convulsions during the newborn period, those with a normal electroencephalogram, taken a few days after the last attack, had an 86 percent chance of normal development by four years of age. On the other hand, a highly abnormal electroencephalogram was always associated with severe motor and mental retardation.

Both the immediate and long-term prognosis for infants who have had seizures during the newborn period is directly related to the cause of the seizures. Thus, a high mortality rate as well as a high incidence of permanent brain damage is associated with massive bleeding into the brain, severe hypoxia (temporary lack of oxygen), or meningitis.

Parents of babies who have had seizures in the few hours or days after birth are, justifiably, concerned not only about their immediate significance but also about what their eventual effect will be on the infant's development. Unfortunately, in too many instances the pediatrician finds himself in a position where he cannot make even an educated guess regarding what is going to happen to the infant in subsequent months. The main reason for the difficulty in making an accurate prognosis regarding either the possibility of seizure recurrence or the likelihood of slow development, is that infants at this early age seldom show very reliable signs or symptoms following a mild to moderate brain injury.

Why is this?

The brain of a newborn infant is an immature organ which functions at a very simple level. We all know that and it is the reason we don't expect too much from a newborn baby. A newborn baby is supposed to cry, eat, swallow, move his extremities at random and in a more or less purposeless manner, urinate, and defecate. And when all his physiologic needs are satisfied, he is supposed to rest or sleep comfortably and quietly. If one stops to think about what a newborn baby can do, the only possible conclusion is that one doesn't need much of what we usually call "brain" to do all these things. Very little, if any, as a matter of fact. Babies born with a condition called hydranencephaly, for example, which is an extreme form of excessive "water" within the brain, have, for all practical purposes, no brain. Nevertheless, as long as the primitive lower part of the brain (brain stem) functions properly, during the first couple of weeks of life they look and behave not a great deal differently from normal babies.

It cannot come as a surprise to anybody, then, that it may not be until a baby is a few months old that the results of a brain injury sustained at the time of birth can become apparent. Because of this, during the first few months of life it is often impossible for pediatricians to predict with any degree of accuracy whether neurologic complications will manifest themselves at a later age. Subsequent examinations of the baby at periodic intervals during the first year of life will almost always clarify any doubts which may exist concerning his development.

My baby had two seizures when he was two days old. I was told that they couldn't find out the cause of them. When I took the baby home, my pediatrician prescribed a medicine which my baby is supposed to take every day for several months and perhaps for a longer time. Will this drug have any effect on my baby's development?

No. Experience with thousands of newborn infants who have received anticonvulsant drugs for months, and sometimes for one or more years after birth, has shown that these medications have no adverse effect on the infant's development. It is understandable that parents may become concerned about their baby's having to take a medicine several times daily for an undetermined period of time. They should rest assured, however, that the daily, continuous administration of anticonvulsants is the only way to prevent the possible recurrence of seizures, and that drugs presently used in the treatment of seizures will not interfere with the mental development of their infant. Furthermore, if the infant remains free of seizures, and no increments in the amount of the daily dosage need to be made, a gradual tapering-off of the drug takes place as he gains weight. As he grows older, he is actually getting less and less medicine even though he is given the same daily dosage. The reason for this is that after anticonvulsant drugs are absorbed in the intestine they are distributed more or less equally throughout all organs of the body, including fat, muscles, and bones. Hence, as the infant puts on weight, a smaller and smaller amount of medicine is actually reaching the brain.

What are the most common causes of seizures after the newborn period?

During the first few years of life, seizures can be due to a number of different causes. In the child of preschool age, the most common type is the so-called febrile seizure, which occurs usually between the ages of six months and two years.

What are febrile seizures?

A febrile seizure has been defined as a convulsion associated with any fever due to infections outside of the brain such as a "strep throat" or an ear infection; as a convulsion precipitated by fever in a patient who has a potential convulsive disorder (epilepsy); or as a generalized grand mal seizure of less than twenty minutes' duration in association with extracerebral (outside the brain) infections, which occurs in a child less than five years of age and in whom a normal electroencephalogram is obtained one week after his temperature has returned to normal. See also page 20 for additional discussion of febrile seizures.

Besides febrile seizures, what are other well-known causes of seizures in young children?

A seizure may be the first symptom of a number of acute illnesses affecting the brain, such as meningitis, encephalitis, intoxications (lead, aspirin, etc.) or bleeding inside the skull. Seizures may also be the initial manifestations or occur at some time during the natural course of uncommon diseases such as brain tumors, congenitally malformed cerebral vessels, or degenerative diseases of the brain. By and large, however, the great majority of children with recurrent seizures do not have or have not previously had any of these diseases.

Secondary or acquired epilepsy is common during the first years of life. Before the age of four, seizures, except febrile seizures, are almost always secondary to some structural abnormality of the brain, or are a consequence of metabolic disturbances such as intermittent lowering of the levels of blood glucose (hypoglycemia) or blood calcium (hypocalcemia). The structural abnormalities that may produce secondary epilepsy at this age of life may be due to a large number of causes, ranging from congenital brain defects and birth injury to extremely rare degenerative diseases of the brain. Primary or idiopathic (unknown cause) epilepsy is rare in the first few years of life, but increases sharply after the age of four.

In more than one way I believe that not being able to determine exactly the cause of a child's epilepsy may be a disguised blessing. It is well known that the possibility that seizures may be the initial manifestation of a serious disease of the brain increases with advancing age. In children, however, seizures are only very rarely the initial symptom of a brain tumor or other chronic and progressive disease affecting the central nervous system. So much for the positive side of the problem.

On the negative side is the fact that in most children with recurrent seizures a cause amenable to specific treatment, such as hypoglycemia, hypocalcemia, lead poisoning, etc., is not found. Nevertheless, all these are diagnostic possibilities that physicians consider and rule out by appropriate studies where the medical history or the results of the physical examination indicates. This is of importance not only because a child who has any of these conditions can be successfully and specifically treated without the need for prolonged therapy with anticonvulsant medications, but also because it enables the physician to exclude a diagnosis of epilepsy.

My four-year-old child had several convulsions between two and three years of age due to episodes of low blood sugar. Why then does he have to take daily an anticonvulsant drug to prevent seizures?

Glucose (sugar) is the human brain's only source of energy. In contrast to other organs, the brain is unable to obtain energy from the burning of fats or proteins. Consequently, its proper functioning depends at all times on a constant and adequate supply of glucose. Repeated and severe episodes of low blood glucose (hypoglycemia), especially when they occur during infancy or early childhood, may produce irreparable damage to a large number of brain cells, the end result being one or more small brain lesions which may become the triggering point of abnormal electrical discharges. Although the original problem is no longer present, it may have produced damage to small portions of the brain, with a subsequent formation of scars from which recurrent seizures may originate.

How can a scar be the source of abnormal electrical brain discharge? Isn't a scar a dead tissue?

Yes, it is. A brain scar, like any other scar, is dead tissue and therefore cannot possibly be the source of anything. However, between the scar proper and the normal surrounding brain there is almost always a layer of brain tissue which is neither totally dead nor entirely normal. It is from these partially damaged areas that epileptic seizures may arise.

How important is severe head trauma as a cause of seizures?

Much more important than is generally recognized. We said in Chapter 1 that children with epilepsy, including those who have grand mal attacks, rarely suffer serious bodily injury as a result of the initial fall during a seizure or as a result of the subsequent jerks of the head or extremities. We will see in a later chapter that this type of blunt head trauma is rarely, if ever, a cause of the worsening of pre-existing epileptic seizures. This is also true of the great majority of head injuries of mild or moderate severity (hard bumps) that children sustain during the course of their everyday activities. They are rarely of any significance.

On the other hand, the number of children who suffer *serious* head injuries and *severe* brain trauma in the United States is very large. Accidents, including those involving a motor vehicle, are the leading cause of death between the ages of one and fourteen years. Nor is that all. Accidents are responsible for more deaths during this period of life than all other causes combined, including cancer (which is second), congenital defects, and infectious diseases.

What can be done to avoid death or serious injury resulting from car accidents?

Everybody knows theoretically what to do to prevent unnecessary fatalities or serious injuries resulting from auto accidents. Yet most of us seem to pay little attention to the problem. During 1972, 56,700 Americans died in automobile accidents and 2 million were maimed. This includes 1,000 car passengers under the age of five and 1,700 between five and fifteen.

It should be remembered that seatbelts and child-restraint devices *do* save lives and that the few seconds we spend buckling up or restraining a child may save us years of pain and remorse. Presently available safety devices have significantly decreased fatal injuries; they also have greatly reduced serious injuries. If you use a shoulder-harness-lap-belt combination, chances are that you will survive just about any collision under sixty miles per hour, and if you don't use it, you can suffer a fatal accident at the ridiculous speed of twelve miles per hour! Mother's lap is certainly not a safe place for small children when riding in a car and standard seatbelts are not safe for small children weighing less than forty pounds. In the last printing of the pamphlet *Stop Risking your Child's Life*, Physicians for Automotive Safety emphasize several aspects related to automobile accidents: "The vast majority of infants and small children riding in automobiles are either inadequately packaged or not restrained at all. Some mothers believe that they can prevent a child sitting beside them from being flung forward by extending their arm in moments of danger. This may be feasible when braking, but it is impossible in a crash. . . . Children over four years of age should be placed on a firm cushion and strapped in with a standard lap belt while sitting upright against the back of the seat."*

In several of its newsletters, Physicians for Automotive Safety also emphasize the need for more safety devices in school buses: "In 1971, 80 children died and 4,200 were injured in school bus accidents." . . . "Injuries could be minimized and death prevented by improved bus design." . . . "Safety features now standard in private cars are absent in school buses, whose design has not undergone significant changes in many decades."

Despite their frequency, accidents involving a motor vehicle are not the main cause of serious bodily injuries in children. It may come as a surprise to many that, in a significant number of children, serious bodily injuries are not the result of accidents or falls, but are due to physical abuse inflicted by the parents.

---

* Information on car restraint devices for children can be obtained by writing to the American Academy of Pediatrics (Council on Child Health), 1801 Hinman Avenue, Evanston, Illinois 60204, or to Physicians for Automotive Safety, 50 Union Avenue, Irvington, New Jersey 07111.

Do you mean that some parents purposefully inflict bodily injury on their children?

Yes, much too often. And the problem is certainly of greater magnitude than the public realizes. Recent statistics show that the incidence of child abuse in this country is increasing and that in all likelihood it will continue to climb before it goes down. Approximately fifty thousand cases of child abuse are reported here every year. The number of non-reported cases is probably several times larger. The death rate among reported cases has been about 4 percent and the rate of permanent injury about 30 percent. The clinical picture of children who have been the victims of parental maltreatment and who have suffered significant bodily injury has been labeled the "battered-child syndrome."

The previously mentioned figures indicate that a large number of young children die each year in this country as a result of injuries inflicted by one or both parents. Worse yet, many of those who survive the "battered-child syndrome" are unfortunately left with permanent brain damage, the least serious of which is probably epileptic seizures.

How can the "battered-child syndrome" be a cause of epilepsy?

In one of several ways. In addition to external evidence of physical abuse (bruises, lacerations, scars, etc.), these children almost always have multiple fractures of the bones of the limbs, chest, and skull. Trauma to the head of the magnitude necessary to cause single or multiple skull fractures can also produce bruising or bleeding inside the brain or on its outer surface where many large cerebral blood vessels are located. Either type of hemorrhage, or bruising of the brain, can destroy portions of the brain and lead eventually to the formation of scars that can become the source of periodic abnormal electrical discharges.

**What are some of the other manifestations of brain damage
seen as a result of the battered-child-syndrome?**

It was mentioned above that epileptic seizures are probably the least serious of brain problems associated with the
battered-child syndrome. Trauma to the brain in infancy and
childhood as a result of child abuse may produce pretty much
the same type of damage observed in association with trauma
to the brain at the time of delivery. The child may be left
with serious neurologic deficits, such as mental retardation,
paralysis on one or both sides of the body, severe behavior
problems, or serious learning difficulties.

**How common are the "uncommon" diseases that may cause
seizures, such as tumors, hemorrhages (strokes), or degenerative diseases of the brain?**

Not common; actually they are so distinctly uncommon
that the word "rare" should probably be used to describe
their frequency. Not that brain tumors do not occur in children. They do. In contrast to what happens in adults, however,
if a child is going to develop a brain tumor, chances are that
the growth will originate from the posterior and inferior parts
of the brain rather than from its anterior and superior portions, which are the regions from which seizures originate.
Seizures, therefore, are rarely the first manifestation of brain
tumors in children and only occur at some time during the
natural course of the disease in less than 5 percent of cases.
Thus, even if a child develops a brain tumor, if and when
seizures finally do occur, many other symptoms will have already been present for a considerable period of time. We can
safely say then that the chances that recurrent epileptic
seizures in a child may represent the initial manifestation of a
brain tumor are very small. The same does not hold true for
adults, especially for those who are forty years of age or older.

With advancing age the risk that seizures may be the first symptom of a brain tumor or other serious condition is several times higher than when seizures begin before the age of twenty.

What about cerebral hemorrhages or strokes? Can children really suffer strokes?

They certainly can. But in children, fortunately, strokes occur even less frequently than brain tumors. In contrast to adults, the most common cause of strokes during infancy and childhood is not hypertension and arteriosclerosis (hardening of the arteries), but congenital defects of the walls of the veins and arteries of the brain, so-called *arteriovenous malformations.* In the past physicians used much more vivid terms to describe these congenital defects, which gave a much clearer picture of their nature. During the past century, for example, physicians referred to such congenital defects as "varicose veins" of the brain and also as "cerebral hemorrhoids." The very thin and fragile walls of the abnormal blood vessels that make up these "varicose veins" not infrequently rupture, producing a brain hemorrhage similar in all respects to that seen in adults with strokes due to hypertension or other causes.

Can arteriovenous malformations of the brain be a cause of seizures before they rupture?

Yes, they can. And not only before, but also at the time they rupture, as well as months or years after the child has recovered from the cerebral hemorrhage. Even though arteriovenous malformations are congenital defects and, therefore, by definition, have been present since birth, rupture seldom occurs before the age of twenty years. Furthermore, if a child is going to have symptoms referable to an arteriovenous malformation of the brain, only in 10 percent of cases will the initial manifestation be recurrent seizures. In the remaining

80 to 90 percent of cases the first symptom will almost always be a stroke.

Can physicians tell by just examining a child when the cause of his seizures is an arteriovenous malformation of the brain?

Not always. Sometimes a diagnosis just on the basis of the medical history and the physical examination may be difficult to make. Several features, however, may suggest that the cause of a child's seizures is a congenital defect of the blood vessels of the brain: (1) seizures due to arteriovenous malformations are almost always focal in nature; they involve only one and almost always the same side of the body. Occasionally the seizure may spread to the other side and develop into a generalized seizure, but only after one side has already been affected for varying periods of time (seconds or minutes); (2) seizures due to arteriovenous malformations of the brain are usually difficult to bring under complete control with anticonvulsant drugs; and (3) the physical examination of an affected child may show the presence of a bruit (murmur) on his head similar to that heard over the chest in patients with congenital heart disease. Thus, if your pediatrician, family physician, or neurologist places his stethoscope on top of your child's head, don't leave his office thinking that he's cracking up and has forgotten where he is supposed to put it. He's only trying to listen for the possible presence of a bruit!

Is there a sure way to find out whether the cause of a child's seizures is a brain tumor or an arteriovenous malformation of the brain?

Yes. At the present time physicians have at their disposal several highly reliable diagnostic techniques to rule out or in the presence of these two conditions. They are called brain scanning, cerebral angiogram, and pneumoencephalogram. The indications for the use of these diagnostic tests as well as a brief description will be given in Chapter 4.

What about degenerative diseases of the brain? What are they, and how often are they the cause of seizures in children?

Degenerative diseases of the brain are groups of conditions having in common a fairly rapid breakdown in the integrity of certain chemical processes going on in the brains of normal people. The exact cause of most of these diseases is either unknown or is still a matter of speculation. In some of them, however, such as Tay-Sachs disease and sulfatide lipidosis, the exact cause of the problem is well established. In these two familial, inherited diseases, researchers have so far demonstrated that there is an absence or a marked decrease in the concentration of a specific brain enzyme which is indispensable for the maintenance of certain vital chemical reactions.

Degenerative diseases of the brain are an even rarer cause of recurrent seizures than brain tumors or arteriovenous malformations. As noted above, most of them are familial, inherited diseases, characterized not only by seizures but also by a rapidly progressive loss of mental faculties, loss of already acquired motor abilities such as walking, loss of manual dexterity, loss of body balance, as well as by a number of other symptoms which are indicative of widespread malfunctioning of the brain. In addition to degenerative diseases of the brain there are a number of inborn errors of metabolism which may produce deterioration of cerebral function.

What can be done if a child has a degenerative brain disease or an inborn error of metabolism that affects the brain?

Unhappily, not a great deal, at least not at the present time. Even though the biochemical defect causing brain deterioration is known for several degenerative diseases of the brain and for many inborn errors of metabolism that may affect the brain, such as phenylketonuria, the treatment of these conditions still remains highly unsatisfactory. In phen-

3. What Other Conditions Can Resemble Epilepsy?

Are there any other conditions that resemble an epileptic attack?

Yes. In more than one respect several well-known disorders can closely resemble an epileptic seizure. Breath-holding spells, during infancy and early childhood, are the most common of these conditions. Sudden loss of consciousness and stiffening of the entire body, for example, which are frequent clinical manifestations of grand mal seizures, are also observed in breath-holding spells. Breath-holding spells can be defined as stereotyped attacks which are characterized by a short period of unconsciousness and abnormal posturing of the body following an unpleasant stimulus or experience such as a fall, spanking, anger, or temper tantrum.

What does it mean to say that breath-holding spells are "stereotyped attacks"?

Breath-holding spells are said to be stereotyped attacks because the sequence of events which take place during the course of different episodes is always the same.

Do you mean that all breath-holding spells are exactly alike?

No. There are two forms of spells, but within each form the sequence of events during a spell is always exactly the same. In the most common form, immediately after a stressful event or a painful stimulus, the child first cries intermittently. A few seconds later his cry becomes sustained and then suddenly he holds his breath at the end of the expiratory (breathing-out) phase of respiration. He then becomes limp, cyanotic (blue-tinged skin) or pale, and loses consciousness. If the attack lasts more than a few seconds, this initial phase is followed by a second one during which there is stiffening or arching of the back. This second phase may or may not be accompanied by a few muscle jerks or flailing movements of the limbs. Occasionally there is incontinence of urine. The phase of stiffening, which usually lasts from ten to twenty seconds, is almost always followed by a phase of limpness.

In the second and much less common type of breath-holding spell, after the child suffers a painful stimulus or an unpleasant experience, he suddenly stops breathing and as a rule becomes limp and unresponsive. He usually remains pale throughout the attack and is less likely to stiffen his body or arch his back.

After a spell the child regains consciousness in a matter of seconds, or, less commonly, falls into a deep sleep. Breath-holding spells usually start between six and twelve months of life, and seldom after the age of four years. About nine out of ten infants with breath-holding spells have their first episode before the age of eighteen months. In very rare instances breath-holding spells may begin after the age of three years.

The frequency of the attacks varies from one child to another. Some may have one episode a month and others as many as five or six per day. Initially they tend to occur at weekly or monthly intervals, reaching a peak frequency of one per week to several per day during the second or third year of life. As the child grows older the spells become less and less frequent.

What causes breath-holding spells?

Nobody knows for certain. The only thing we know for sure is that they are always brought on by some kind of unpleasant or frustrating experience or by a painful stimulus. In contrast to true epileptic attacks, breath-holding spells never come out of the blue.

When do children "outgrow" breath-holding spells?

Ninety percent of children with breath-holding spells stop having them by six years of age or before, the remaining 10 percent by age seven. For some obscure reason breath-holding spells appear to run in families. In one large series of children a group of researchers found that in 30 percent of them there was a history of similar attacks in other members of the family.

Do children with breath-holding spells have any special problems when they grow older?

Special maybe, but certainly not serious. Several investigators have commented on the high incidence of fainting spells or syncopal attacks brought on by pain or anger when these children get older. The outlook in terms of mental development or the possible occurrence of convulsive seizures (epilepsy) is excellent. Neither mental retardation nor epilepsy are more common in children with breath-holding spells than in the general population.

How do breath-holding spells differ from epileptic attacks?

In several ways. Because of the above-mentioned clinical characteristics of breath-holding spells, they can only be confused with grand mal seizures. Breath-holding spells can be differentiated from grand mal seizures by (1) the constant presence of an immediately precipitating stimulus (fall, anger, etc.), (2) the stereotyped sequence of events that take place during attacks, and (3) the frequent lack of drowsiness or sleepiness following the spell, which is almost always seen after a grand mal seizure. Arching of the back, a common manifestation of breath-holding spells, is rarely if ever seen in true epileptic seizures. In addition, in contrast to patients with epilepsy, the electroencephalogram is normal in children with breath-holding spells.

In spite of all these differentiating features a diagnosis of breath-holding spells may sometimes be quite difficult to make, especially in those cases which are not preceded by the child's crying. Spells that appear very similar may be true epileptic seizures, or may be attacks of syncope (fainting) due to diseases of the heart or other organs. In rare instances a child may have grand mal seizures, with or without associated convulsive movements, which are always precipitated by a painful stimulus. We must emphasize, then, the need for a thorough examination by a physician in all cases in which a child loses consciousness—including those instances in which this is preceded by crying. We believe that in most instances, and especially if parents are good observers and better historians, the differentiation between breath-holding spells and grand mal seizures is not difficult to make.

There are several important reasons why it is imperative that an accurate differentiation be made, if at all possible, in all cases. Breath-holding spells are a common problem in early childhood. If a complete and exact history of the attacks is not elicited from the parents, the physician may end up treating the patient as if he had grand mal seizures and unnecessarily prescribing phenobarbital or some other anticonvulsant drug for three or more years. And if the patient is erroneously labeled as having epilepsy, unnecessary damage can be done to the family as well as the child. Even though the child will spontaneously stop having breath-holding spells when he reaches the age of five or six years, there is no easy way to erase a diagnosis of epilepsy entered into the patient's record. Information from these records may be requested at a later age by the department of motor vehicles, employers, or insurance companies. Since biases and prejudices are still quite prevalent among the general population, it is not difficult to see that a long-lasting disservice to the child can be done if a distinction between breath-holding spells and epilepsy is not made.

Can breath-holding spells interfere with the mental development of the child?

No. Long-term follow-up of twenty or more years of large numbers of children who have had breath-holding spells during early childhood has shown that, irrespective of the frequency or severity of the attacks, they do not interfere with the mental development of the child. In this regard it is of interest to note that the overwhelming majority of children who have breath-holding spells are of average or above-average intelligence. Although an occasional case has been reported by other physicians, I have never personally seen breath-holding spells in a child who was moderately or severely mentally retarded.

What can be done to prevent the occurrence of breath-holding spells?

Not a great deal. A number of drugs have been used unsuccessfully in the past to prevent the recurrence of breath-holding spells. I mentioned above that the child with breath-holding spells is almost always bright. More often than not he is also an overprotected and manipulative child who seeks instant gratification of everything he wants. When physicians reassure the parents of these children that the attacks are not dangerous, the parent can act with greater confidence, treat the child like any other "normal" child, and avoid overprotecting him. Understandably, the parents of a child with a history of attacks tend to give in to his whims in an attempt to avoid provoking anger or temper tantrums which may precipitate an attack. If at all possible, a calm and matter-of-fact attitude on the part of the parents at the time of subsequent spells will, in the great majority of instances, help to reinforce in the child the feeling that the spells are not an effective way of manipulating his parents or his environment.

What else may resemble epilepsy?

Another condition that may closely resemble an epileptic seizure is fainting or syncope. Syncope is the temporary loss of consciousness secondary to a transient decrease in the amount of blood reaching the brain. This may occur as a result of extreme fatigue, prolonged standing in a hot environment, getting up after prolonged bed rest, or with a sudden change of the body from the horizontal to the erect position, severe pain, anemia, and, not infrequently, just the sight of blood or other psychologic or emotional stress. Immediately before losing consciousness the person feels weak and light-headed and breaks out in a cold sweat. Within seconds there is blurring of vision or total blindness followed by loss of consciousness, which as a rule lasts from a few seconds to one minute. During a fainting spell or syncope the individual is pale, has clammy skin, a slow pulse, and low blood pressure. If the attack lasts longer than one minute, jerking motions of the arms and legs or loss of bladder or bowel control can occur.

In a young child it may sometimes be difficult to differentiate simple syncope from an epileptic seizure which is not associated with convulsive movements. In most instances, syncope can be differentiated from epileptic seizures by the almost constant presence of warning signs. Ordinary fainting spells rarely, if ever, come out of the blue. For a few seconds before losing consciousness the person knows that he may faint and after recovery he remembers what has happened to him. Syncope occurs with greater frequency in adults than in children.

Can children consciously or subconsciously fake an epileptic seizure?

They certainly can. Still, at least in our experience, this is not a very frequent occurrence. Why in heaven should a child do a thing like that? In most cases it is an excellent way by which a child can manipulate his environment. In our experience the most common form of hysterical manifestation which may resemble an epileptic seizure occurs in teen-aged girls who complain of periodic and vague episodes of dizziness and a feeling of general weakness or fatigue that sometimes leads to what appears to be a fainting spell. Afterward these children will often say that, although during the episode they could hear the voices from people around them, somehow they were unable to answer questions or to utter a single word. Sometimes telling this type of spell apart from psychomotor seizures can be extremely difficult even for the shrewdest of physicians. A detailed description of the episodes, and especially of the circumstances preceding them, can be invaluable information to the physician confronted with this dilemma.

Infants and young children, of course, can hardly be expected to have sufficient intellectual ability to pull one of these tricks successfully. The situation is entirely different in older children. And more so, and for reasons which are not completely clear, if the child is a girl between the ages of twelve and sixteen years.

How can one differentiate a true epileptic seizure from a hysterical attack?

This is not an easy question to answer, and therefore I will make no attempt to give a magic formula with which parents might be able to tell them apart. As a matter of fact, I have none. It is the physician's role and responsibility to evaluate each individual child and pass judgment on the basis of a painstaking history of the episodes as well as the information provided by the physical examination (if possible at the time of an episode), and pertinent laboratory tests. Since a detailed history of the attacks is by far the most important piece of information on which the physician can make a decision regarding their true nature, we must emphasize that parents should keep exact track of what happens to the child before and during the entire episode. Grand mal attacks are extremely difficult to fake. So far we have seen only two or three children who attempted to reproduce them but with very little success. Children who attempt to imitate a grand mal seizure will usually thrash around and perform more or less purposeful muscle movements with their arms, legs, and eyes. The true stiffness of the body, which is almost always the first manifestation of a grand mal attack, and the brief, strong, and purposeless muscle jerks of the limbs are extremely hard, if not impossible, to reproduce. As would be expected, these children do not bite their tongues, and seldom if ever have urinary or fecal incontinence. In most cases, therefore, physicians have little difficulty in differentiating a hysterical attack from a true epileptic seizure. Of course this is true only in those instances in which the physician can witness one of the attacks. On the other hand, the differentiation between a hysterical attack and a true epileptic seizure only on the basis of the information provided by the parents may be a very difficult diagnostic problem.

The onset of a hysterical attack is almost always less sudden than that of a true epileptic seizure, and in most instances bodily injury does not occur as a consequence of the spell. As we will see later, in most patients with epilepsy the electroencephalogram shows some type of abnormal waves. In children with hysterical seizures, it is normal. If an electroencephalogram is performed on a hysterical child during the course of an attack or immediately thereafter, it shows normal brain waves, whereas the electroencephalogram recorded during an epileptic seizure reveals continuous "spiky" waves and very slow, high-amplitude waves after the seizure has subsided.

In summary, differentiating between faked and true epileptic seizures may not be an easy thing to do and can seriously tax the ingenuity of the physician. Furthermore, if hysterical or malingered attacks develop in a child who previously had true epileptic seizures, this differentiation will be much more difficult to make.

Is it possible to confuse unconsciousness due to head trauma with that caused by an epileptic attack?

Seldom. Since in the vast majority of instances there is external evidence of head injury in the form of scalp lacerations or bruises, a diagnosis of sudden loss of consciousness secondary to head trauma only rarely presents any difficulties. Occasionally, however, it is very difficult, even for physicians, to determine whether loss of consciousness is due to head trauma or whether the head trauma is secondary to a fall at the onset of an epileptic attack.

In addition to head trauma and epilepsy there are a number of other conditions which may also be a cause of loss of consciousness: intoxications, diabetic coma, and infections of the brain or of its covering membranes. We don't need to emphasize, then, that it is mandatory that any child who is seen to lose consciousness or who is found unconscious should be immediately evaluated by a physician.

Can children suffer from heart conditions which may resemble an epileptic attack?

Yes, they can. But children rarely suffer from heart attacks. Sudden attacks of dizziness or temporary loss of consciousness may sometimes occur as the result of a complete block of the electrical waves going from one to another chamber of the heart. As a consequence of this electrical block there is a sudden and marked slowing in the rate of the heartbeat and a decrease in the heart's output of blood which results in a transient impairment of brain circulation and a sudden and brief loss of consciousness. When complete heart block occurs in children, it is usually a congenital defect; that is to say it is present at birth, and seldom causes any problems. On the other hand, children with congenital narrowing of one of the heart valves (aortic stenosis) are notoriously prone to attacks of syncope, which also appear to be related to decreased cardiac output of blood and temporary impairment in the amount of blood reaching the brain.

What about drug addiction?

Nowadays this is certainly a distinct possibility, especially among teen-agers. In the past couple of years we have erroneously made a diagnosis of psychomotor seizures in at least two adolescents who underwent attacks which were characterized by marked mental confusion or irrational behavior and who later admitted taking drugs before the time of the attacks.

Can nightmares or sleepwalking be confused with epilepsy?

Yes, in rare instances, either one of these conditions can be mistaken for psychomotor seizures. If what appears to be a nightmare or an episode of night terror is indeed a psychomotor seizure, it is more than likely that the child will also have similar episodes during the daytime. In addition, the electroencephalogram is normal in children with nightmares or episodes of sleepwalking and is abnormal in the great majority of those suffering from psychomotor seizures.

What about bedwetting?

In a child with a well-documented history of grand mal seizures, an isolated occurrence of bedwetting may be the only evidence that a child has had an epileptic attack during the night. Repeated episodes of bedwetting alone in a child who has already achieved bladder control during the daytime is due to causes other than epilepsy.

Bedwetting (enuresis) in children is a very common problem. Approximately 15 to 20 percent of children between the ages of six and thirteen years seen for routine medical examinations are affected.

What causes enuresis?

There is no single answer to this question. In some children the cause of enuresis may be a psychological or emotional problem. Not uncommonly, however, the reverse is true; behavior problems which these children may have are the result of enuresis rather than their cause. In other children enuresis is a manifestation of their inability to learn to control urination during a critical period of development as a result of small bladder capacity.

In rare cases enuresis may be due to abnormalities of the urologic tract or to lesions of the lower part of the spinal cord. When this is the case, the child will almost always have trouble with urination during the day as well as during the night.

Is there anything else that can be confused with an epileptic seizure?

Yes. No matter how difficult it may be to believe, masturbation in a young child can be confused with epileptic attacks or with episodes of low blood sugar (hypoglycemia).

In Chapter 1 we mentioned that in ancient Greece, sexual

excesses and sexual aberrations were thought to be one of the many causes responsible for seizures. For more than two thousand years, masturbation, especially when practiced during childhood and adolescence, remained in the mind of laymen as well as physicians a well-established cause of seizures. Sir William Gowers, eminent English neurologist, wrote in 1885 in his book on epilepsy:

Many circumstances rendered it very difficult to determine the influence of masturbation as the cause of epilepsy. The habit is common in epileptic boys, as in others, but we cannot infer that, in all such cases, it is the cause of the disease. The etiological [causal] relation can only be regarded as established when the arrest of the habit as by circumcision arrests the disease. I have so frequently in boys met with this form of attack in association with the practice of masturbation, that I can scarcely doubt their etiological connection.

In another chapter of the same book Dr. Gowers states in reference to a thirteen-year-old boy who suffered from a peculiar type of seizure: "He had twelve or fourteen fits a day on various treatments. It was then found that he practiced masturbation; a blister on the prepuce reduced the fits to two from seven daily. He was then circumcised and the attacks ceased at once and did not recur." It is not unlikely that Dr. Gowers' young patient did not suffer from epileptic seizures but that he repeatedly practiced masturbation, and that the external manifestations of his orgasms were mistaken for epileptic attacks.

During the past few years we have seen several young children who were referred to our seizure clinic with a diagnosis of epileptic seizures because of periodic episodes which consisted of staring spells, flushing of the face, and profuse sweating of the forehead, followed in a matter of seconds by pallor of the face and total relaxation of the body, the child remaining for a few seconds afterward in a state of generalized limpness and seemingly unresponsive. After careful observation of subsequent episodes the parents of these children reported to us that all the episodes occurred while the child was sitting or lying on his back with his legs drawn up on his abdomen, and only after he had vigorously rubbed his thighs together, thereby stimulating his genitalia.

As pointed out by Dr. Gowers as early as 1885, masturbation in children is a common and, we may add today, in the great majority of instances a harmless practice. Nevertheless, for many years masturbation was held responsible for a variety of illnesses, such as tuberculosis, loss of memory, feeblemindedness and other physical as well as psychiatric illnesses. Since nowadays it is a well-established fact that masturbation is an almost universal practice in boys and a common occurrence in girls, if the habit were indeed responsible for epilepsy, there would be very few nonepileptics left in this world.

Can nervous tics be confused with focal motor seizures which are characterized not by loss of consciousness but only by sudden jerks of one side of the body, one limb or one side of the mouth or face?

Hardly. Nervous tics, or "habit spasms" as physicians call them, are stereotyped movements of a group of muscles repeated at variable intervals and occurring in a background of complete normality. The sudden movements of habit spasms, in contrast to *any* type of epileptic seizure, always follow the same pattern with regard to such variables as rhythm, intensity, amplitude and duration. The repetitive movements of habit spasms may manifest as facial grimaces, winking, shrugging of one or both shoulders, or mild extension of the head and retraction of the jaw.

In this context we should mention that at least once or twice a year we see children suffering from Sydenham's chorea (St. Vitus dance) who have previously been diagnosed and referred to us as epileptics. Sydenham's chorea is one of the many forms in which rheumatic fever may manifest itself. Since the advent of effective antibiotic therapy for the treatment of "strep throat" and other "strep" infections (the underlying cause of rheumatic fever), its incidence has decreased considerably. More than 75 percent of cases occur between the age of five and fifteen years. Females are affected twice as frequently as males. Sydenham's chorea or St. Vitus dance is characterized by the sudden appearance of involuntary, brief, and explosive movements of variable amplitude involving the extremities, face, and tongue in a previously healthy child. Because of the abnormal involuntary movements, patients with Sydenham's chorea may have great difficulty in walking, feeding themselves, or talking. Sydenham's chorea is a self-limited disease. An episode rarely lasts more than three months. Throughout the duration of the episode, and in spite of the marked physical disability brought about by the involuntary movements, there is no loss of awareness or loss of consciousness.

4. Diagnosing Epilepsy

Is it easy to make a diagnosis of epilepsy?

Usually, but not always. It is quite obvious that even the most inexperienced of observers may recognize a grand mal seizure. One doesn't have to be a physician to tell that somebody who suddenly loses consciousness, falls to the ground, and has violent muscle jerks of one or more limbs is having a convulsion. However, we should remember that about 30 percent of children with epilepsy suffer from recurrent spells which are entirely different from that which in the minds of most people is associated with epilepsy. In this context I should repeat here that *not all shaking spells are epilepsy and many nonshaking spells are.* I also discussed in Chapter 2 several conditions in which a child may have recurrent grand mal seizures and yet not suffer from epilepsy. To complicate things even further, several other disorders occur, especially in early childhood, which may closely resemble epileptic seizures (Chapter 3).

How do physicians make a diagnosis of epilepsy?

The most reliable and important item in the diagnosis of any type of epilepsy is the history of the attacks. By taking an accurate and as complete as possible a history, physicians are, in the great majority of cases, in a position to differentiate true epileptic seizures from other conditions that closely resemble them. By the same token, for an accurate categorization of the type of seizures a child is having, there is no substitute for a detailed and precise history of the attacks. This is particularly important in those children whose seizures are not accompanied by loss of consciousness or obvious jerking of one or more extremities. It is important, then, that parents make an effort to recall exactly what happens to the child from the beginning to the very end of an attack. It is also helpful to physicians if parents are able to remember what took place before or immediately after an episode. What was the child doing at the time? Was he hurt prior to the onset of the seizure? Did he cry for a few seconds and then hold his breath and arch his back? Did he suddenly fall to the floor without any apparent reason and recover in a matter of seconds? Was he watching a defective TV set at the time he suddenly had an unexplained fluttering of his eyelids and a few twitches around his mouth? Was he drowsy immediately after an attack? Did he urinate or did he have a bowel movement during the spell? Loss of bladder control with involuntary urination is not uncommon in patients who suffer from minor motor seizures which closely resemble petit mal. A single piece of information such as this, for example, may help the physician in making an accurate diagnosis as to the type of seizures the child is having and enable him to institute the appropriate treatment.

Most parents are unaware of how important an accurate description of the seizure is for the physician, so that he can tell what is and what is not an epileptic attack and can then be able to categorize accurately a particular type of seizure. Under the stress and panic of a grand mal seizure, most parents will not be able to sort out relevant from irrelevant observations, and are likely to describe the episode in a sentence or two, then go on to how upset everybody was, what each member of the family attempted to do to stop the attack, etc., etc. My personal impression is that the great majority of parents are very poor observers under these circumstances and, foremost, extremely poor at estimating time. It should be admitted that the unexpected occurrence of a grand mal seizure in a family member is a dramatic and frightening experience. Nobody can expect parents not to lose their grasp of time when they are suddenly confronted with such an experience. Yet we should also remember that about 30 percent of children with epilepsy have seizures which are not really very dramatic experiences. I never cease to be amazed, for example, at the ease with which parents confuse seconds with minutes and sometimes minutes with hours. I said in Chapter 1 that petit mal seizures, which are characterized by very brief lapses of awareness, never last more than twenty to thirty seconds and more often than not last only from five to ten. In spite of this, when parents are asked about the duration of the attacks they will often state that they last anywhere from one to two minutes. Now, in the case of grand mal seizures it doesn't actually make much difference from a diagnostic standpoint whether the seizure lasted forty-five seconds or fifteen minutes. There is really no way that a physician can fail to give it its proper name. But, in the case of other types of seizures, the duration of the attack can be a crucial factor on which to base an accurate diagnosis. For example, if the seizures *really* last one to two minutes, the physician can be certain that your child is not having petit mal, myoclonic, or akinetic seizures, but some other type of attacks.

Besides a detailed and accurate history of the attacks, what else can be done to find out the cause of seizures?

It is almost superfluous to mention that, in addition to an accurate description of the attacks, the evaluation of a child with seizures should also include a detailed history of the mother's pregnancy, labor, and delivery, all his previous illnesses (including severe head trauma), an inquiry into the family history for seizures or related problems, a summary of his main milestones of motor and mental development, and a complete physical examination. Yet, when all possible relevant information is put together, physicians cannot help but be surprised, and often frustrated, at the large number of children with epilepsy in whom nothing can be uncovered as the probable cause for their difficulties. In the great majority of children with seizures the physical examination, for example, is of little value in making a diagnostic assumption of the cause of their seizures. And, with the exception of the electroencephalogram, I must say that the same is also true of most laboratory tests. In an occasional case, however, the physician may find that the cause of a child's grand mal seizures is a temporary lowering of the levels of blood glucose or a persistent lowering of the levels of blood calcium. Since changes in the blood concentration of these compounds may give rise to recurrent seizures which are impossible to distinguish from true epileptic seizures, physicians routinely perform blood determinations of these substances as part of the initial evaluation of a child with seizures. A single normal blood level of calcium can rule out hypocalcemia. The same, however, is not true of hypoglycemia. We said above that the lowering of the blood levels of glucose can be transitory. Therefore, a determination done days after a seizure can be normal. At any rate, if the physician strongly suspects a diagnosis of hypoglycemia, he can do additional tests that will confirm or rule out this possibility.

Parents of epileptic children are also aware that as part of the initial evaluation of a child with seizures, physicians usually request x-rays of the skull and, in practically all cases, an electroencephalogram (brain-wave test).

How can x-rays of the skull be of importance in finding out the cause of a child's seizures?

In fewer ways than most parents seem to believe. Great misconceptions regarding the diagnostic value of x-rays of the skull exist among laymen. Most parents of epileptic children appear to expect a great deal more than is warranted from this diagnostic test. Actually, x-ray examination of the skull in children with seizures is of limited diagnostic value. Only the bones of the skull and the bones of the face show up in such x-rays. Neither the brain proper nor other structures inside the skull can be visualized by this technique. But in a very small number of patients with epilepsy x-ray examination of the skull may reveal the presence of areas of calcification within the brain. When calcium, which is a radiopaque substance, has accumulated in one or more areas of the brain, skull x-rays can show something that may give the physician a clue as to the possible cause of a child's seizures. For example, certain infections which the baby may acquire during intrauterine life may infect the brain and produce many small areas of calcification under its surface or around the cavities (ventricles) normally present in its center. Yet intrauterine infections of the brain account for a very small percentage of cases of epilepsy in children. Also rarely, skull x-rays may show an area of calcification inside a brain tumor or inside congenitally malformed blood vessels (arteriovenous malformations) within the substance of the brain. As noted in an earlier chapter, lesions such as these, at least in children, are very rare causes of recurrent seizures in childhood.

In summary, x-ray examination of the skull is normal in the overwhelming majority of epileptic children. I should stress here that all this means is that the bony case surrounding the brain shows no abnormalities and that within the substance of the brain there are no areas of increased density (calcifications). Parents of epileptic children should know, then, that x-ray examination of the skull is, more often than not, an unrewarding diagnostic test. It will seldom tell the physician the cause of a child's seizures. Yet, since there is no way of knowing in advance the child in whom skull x-rays *will* reveal something of importance, physicians have no choice but to perform the test in just about all children with seizures, irrespective of what the clinical history and the physical examination may show.

What about the electroencephalogram or brain-wave test?

In contrast to x-rays of the skull, the electroencephalogram or brain-wave test is an important test in the diagnosis as well as the treatment of epilepsy. Nevertheless, as we will soon see, like any other diagnostic technique, it also has its limitations.

"Electroencephalogram" is a word put together from three others meaning "electric brain writing." The electroencephalogram, also called EEG, is the recording, on a running band of paper, of the electrical activity generated by approximately two-thirds of the surface of the brain. Small disc electrodes, which are applied to the scalp and held in place by a special adhesive material, pick up this electrical activity. Fine wires run from the electrodes to a machine called an electroencephalograph, which picks up and amplifies the low-voltage electrical discharges generated by the surface of the brain. These amplified currents move pen writers on a moving band of paper, and the tracings on this paper are a record of the brain waves of the patient.

The recording of the electrical brain waves is an entirely safe and painless procedure. Depending on the age of the child, it can be performed with the patient sitting on a reclining chair or lying down on a bed. The record on paper is a series of long, wavy lines, one line for each section of the brain underlying the area where the electrodes are applied.

An electroencephalogram varies considerably from one person to another. It also changes with age. During infancy the electroencephalogram shows mostly from three to six waves per second. As the child gets older the frequency of the brain waves increases, the adult pattern of about nine to ten waves per second being reached at age fourteen.

The electroencephalograph, an extremely sensitive machine, increases the amplitude of the electrical activity of the brain about a million times before it is recorded. Because of this great sensitivity, any movements of the muscles of the face, forehead, scalp, or eyeballs will also be picked up. Thus, a number of nonbrain electrical discharges will be introduced into the recording which will overlap with and can make the true brain waves difficult to interpret. Therefore, although the electroencephalogram is an entirely painless and harmless test, it does require a certain degree of cooperation on the part of the patient.

What then about doing an electroencephalogram in infants or in uncooperative young children?

In most instances a well-trained and patient EEG technician will have no difficulties in obtaining a record which will be of sufficiently good quality to be a reasonably good sample of the electrical activity of the brain during a twenty- to thirty-minute period. If a child is too young to cooperate or if he is hyperactive, he can be sedated and the recording performed while he is asleep. Although the electroencephalogram changes somewhat during natural sleep or during sleep artificially induced by drugs, the physician is nevertheless still able to obtain reliable information from it.

Why don't physicians perform the actual test?

For two reasons: it is time-consuming and, actually, it does not require a physician's skill to do it. EEG technicians are well-trained individuals who have received at least two

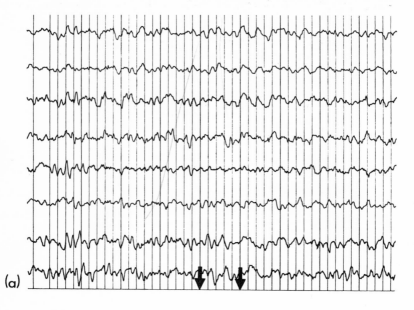

(a)

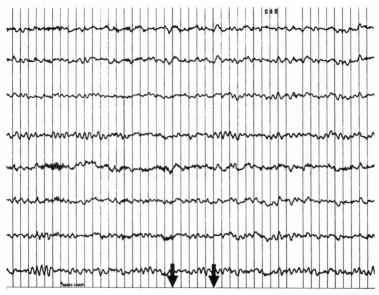

(b)

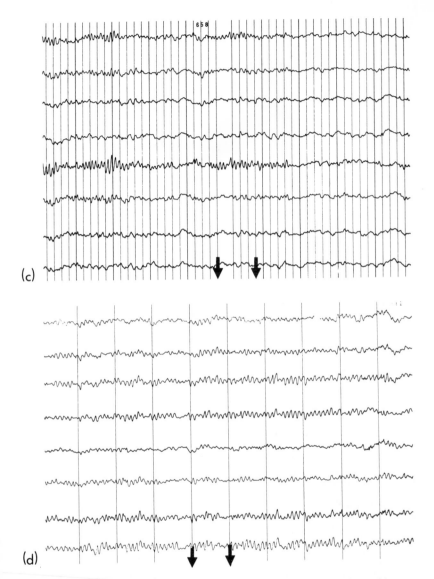

Fig. 2. Normal electroencephalogram at age one (a), age four (b), age ten (c) and age fourteen (d). One second of recording is indicated between arrows. There is a predominance of slow waves of about four per second in tracing at age one year. With advancing age the frequency of predominant waves increases to about nine to ten per second. Also notice that tracing becomes much more regular and uniform as a child gets older.

years of training in their specialty. They are thus in a position to do as good a job as the technician who takes an x-ray of your broken leg or the technician who takes your electrocardiogram.

Who interprets the electroencephalogram?

The interpretation or reading of an electroencephalogram is usually done by a neurologist or other physician who has received specialized training.

How valuable is the electroencephalogram as a diagnostic test in children with seizures?

The electroencephalogram is a very useful diagnostic tool in children with seizures. Yet we should emphasize that, contrary to popular belief, its value is restricted in the great majority of cases to the presence or absence of electrical seizure activity; the electroencephalogram cannot tell the physician what parents are usually anxious to know: what is the cause of the seizures.

As noted earlier, the electroencephalogram is normal in individuals with hysterical or malingered attacks. By the same token the electroencephalogram is helpful in differentiating psychomotor seizures from episodes of strange or bizarre behavior. For example, sometimes a child may have suffered an unusual episode of abnormal behavior while in strange surroundings, while in the presence of unreliable observers, or when his parents or other family members have not had a chance to witness the episode from beginning to end. In such cases, the electroencephalogram can provide the physician with invaluable information regarding the true nature of the attack.

Certain forms of abnormal electrical brain activity recorded by the electroencephalogram are more or less specific for certain type of seizures. Consequently, the electroencephalogram can also help the prescribing physician in the selection of the anticonvulsant drug most likely to benefit the child. This is especially true in young children in whom the history of the attacks is sometimes not sufficient for physicians to tell what type of seizures a child is having.

What is an abnormal electroencephalogram?

When we say that an electroencephalogram is abnormal what we mean is simply that the brain waves are different from those observed in normal individuals. However, in children with epilepsy the abnormal brain waves do not necessarily have to be present during the entire twenty or thirty minutes of the recording. As happens with seizures, which are intermittent phenomena, the abnormalities seen in the electroencephalogram of epileptics occur also intermittently and take the form of short bursts of abnormal waves on a more or less normal background. Epileptic brain waves can be differentiated from normal ones by changes in their frequency, size, and shape. The abnormalities seen in the electroencephalogram of epileptics may vary from nonspecific changes in one or more areas of the brain to changes which are more or less specific for a particular type of seizure.

Do all children with seizures have an abnormal electroencephalogram?

No. An abnormal electroencephalogram is seen in approximately 70 to 85 percent of children with a history of seizures. I mentioned earlier that the electroencephalogram surveys only about two-thirds of the electrical activity of the surface of the brain. Because of the distance which exists between the pickup electrodes on the scalp and the surface of the brain, and because of the electrodes' location in relation to deep portions of the brain, the electrical activity of at least one-third of the brain surface and that of all other under-

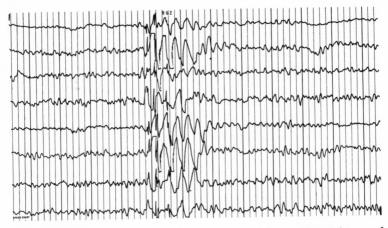

Fig. 3. Electroencephalogram in a five-year-old boy with a history of grand mal seizures. Notice burst of electrical seizure discharge in the center of the photograph, lasting approximately one second and interrupting an otherwise normal record. The electrical seizure discharge was not accompanied by any external manifestation of seizure.

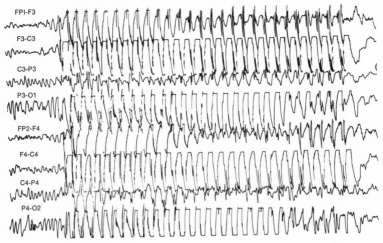

Fig. 4. Electroencephalogram of ten-year-old girl demonstrating diffuse burst of spike and wave activity during a petit mal attack. Both the seizure and the abnormal wave rhythm lasted about seven seconds.

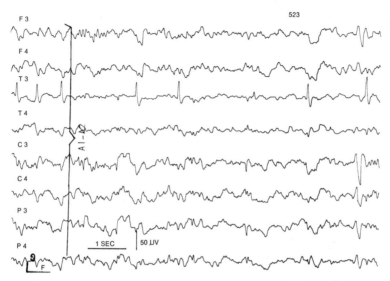

Fig. 5. Electroencephalogram in five-year-old child with psychomotor seizures, showing several very sharp waves (spikes) in left temporal region (T3).

lying areas cannot be recorded. It is not surprising then that in about one out of four epileptic children the electroencephalogram is either normal or shows only minor changes which can also be observed in people who have never had seizures. In extremely rare instances the electroencephalogram can even be normal while the patient is actually having a seizure. Moreover, the electroencephalogram represents only the recording of the electrical behavior of the brain during a twenty- to thirty-minute period. In contrast to the electrocardiogram (the recording of the electrical activity of the heart), which is a repetitive and more or less monotonous phenomenon, the electroencephalogram is a sample of only a brief period of the constantly changing electrical activity of the brain.

Should all children with seizures have an electroencephalogram?

Yes. And not only as part of their initial evaluation, but also at periodic intervals later on to determine the effects of therapy on any abnormal electrical activity which might have been present prior to the initiation of treatment. If a patient's seizures are well controlled, most physicians recommend repeating the electroencephalogram at yearly intervals. If seizures are difficult to control, the physician may find it necessary to repeat the test at more frequent intervals.

Do the abnormal waves seen in the electroencephalogram of epileptic children improve with anticonvulsant treatment?

Yes. In the great majority of cases any abnormal findings which may have been present in the electroencephalogram prior to the initiation of treatment will disappear after the child has been free of seizures for two, three, or more years. Occasionally, however, the electroencephalogram may show signs of improvement in spite of the fact that the child is still having seizures. Several factors can explain this paradoxical situation. For one thing, in a certain number of epileptic children, especially those who have had an occasional grand mal seizure, the electroencephalogram may have been entirely normal or may have shown only minor changes before the beginning of anticonvulsant therapy. In addition, since the electroencephalogram represents the recording of the electrical activity of the brain during a period of only twenty to thirty minutes, it is always possible that by mere chance no abnormalities can be demonstrated during this relatively short span.

Should anticonvulsant medications be discontinued before doing an electroencephalogram?

Over the years I have known a number of physicians who advise parents to take a child with seizures off his anticon-

vulsant medications for twenty-four or forty-eight hours before an electroencephalogram is performed. I believe that
this is a totally unjustified policy. For one thing, if a child
has had one or more seizures he will have to be treated for
a prolonged period of time irrespective of what the electroencephalogram shows or doesn't show. And 15 to 30 percent
of children with epilepsy have a normal electroencephalogram
even when they are not taking medicines. As happens with
many other medical conditions, a diagnosis of epilepsy is
made primarily on the basis of the clinical history and not on
the basis of a test. Moreover, the changes in the brain waves
produced by anticonvulsant drugs are well known to physicians who interpret electroencephalograms. Parents may ask
themselves, "What if the anticonvulsant drugs suppresses the
evidence of epilepsy in the electroencephalogram?" Actually,
it doesn't make any difference. The more and the earlier abnormal brain waves are suppressed, the better. As we will
later see, a child with seizures will have to receive anticonvulsant medications for a prolonged period of time, whether
his electroencephalogram is normal or abnormal. And sudden
withdrawal of anticonvulsant medications, especially if they
have been taken for a prolonged period of time is certainly
the best way to bring on a seizure. Thus, unless your physician
has specifically instructed you to discontinue anticonvulsants,
please don't do it on your own.

**Can the electroencephalogram show what part of the brain is
not functioning properly?**

In many cases of epilepsy the electroencephalogram may
reveal that a certain part of the brain is intermittently sending abnormal electrical discharges. For example, in a number
of children with grand mal seizures it shows that the abnormal discharges are coming from a fairly discrete portion
of the brain surface that controls movements, and, in children
with psychomotor seizures, that these have their origin in the

lateral aspect of the brain surface (temporal lobes), almost directly overlying the region of the ear. In patients with petit mal who are not receiving anticonvulsant treatment, the electroencephalogram almost always shows typical bursts of spike and wave complexes occurring at the same time over the entire surface of the brain. In a large percentage of epileptic children, however, the electroencephalogram shows that two or more areas of the brain are producing periodic bursts of abnormal electrical activity. Children with myoclonic and akinetic seizures, for example, often have electroencephalograms which show abnormal wave patterns in more than one single area of the brain.

In summary, the electroencephalogram is doubtless a very useful tool in the diagnosis and management of children with seizures. It is, however, as is the case with many other laboratory tests, a limited technique which will answer only some of the questions the physician would like to ask, and much too often almost none of the questions parents are asking. Parents are primarily interested in knowing what the cause of their child's seizures is. They are also naturally anxious to know whether or not the "brain-wave test" shows any evidence of brain damage. At best the electroencephalogram can suggest in some cases the likelihood that the cause of a child's seizures is a small atrophic lesion (scar) in a certain part of the brain's surface. It cannot, however, tell physicians what the cause of the scar is.

Foremost in the minds of parents is the question "Can the electroencephalogram tell how well our child will do in terms of mental development?" For reasons which are difficult to explain, the value of the electroencephalogram as an index of a child's intelligence, and as a prognosticator of future mental development, has been greatly overemphasized. This has occurred, unfortunately, not only in regard to patients with epilepsy but also in those with mental retardation. Parents ought to remember—as we have already stated—that the electroencephalogram surveys the electrical activity of only about two-thirds of the surface of the brain. It is obvious then that it cannot possibly provide information concerning what is going on in the rest of the brain. And, even if it did, the electrical activity of the brain recorded by the electroencephalogram has nothing to do with a person's intelligence, imagination, ability to learn, or anything else relating to mental abilities. Consequently, the electroencephalogram is a test which cannot tell physicians or psychologists how intelligent a child is, how retarded he may eventually be, and, if a child is retarded, how fast his progress will be in the future or what is he going to be like five or ten years from now. You can be sure that, if the electroencephalogram were able to answer this type of questions, psychologists would have been run out of business long ago. For a proper answer to questions such as these, there is no substitute for a careful evaluation of a child's progress over a certain period of time, or a formal evaluation of his intellectual abilities, by a psychologist, when he is old enough to cooperate. What I just said underscores the relevance of what I always like to tell the worried parents of children who have abnormal electroencephalograms. I tell them that, as far as I know, it is far better to have a child with an abnormal electroencephalogram and normal mental development than a child who has a normal electroencephalogram but who is "slow" when compared with other children of his same age. This is just another way of saying that the electroencephalogram has little to do with intelligence.

To sum up, the electroencephalogram is a useful diagnostic test in children with epilepsy, but like any other test has its own built-in limitations. I should re-emphasize that it is unrealistic to expect from a laboratory test answers to questions which it cannot possibly provide. To delude oneself into believing that the electroencephalogram will shed light on any of the previously mentioned matters is no more realistic than to expect peaches from an apple tree. Unhappily, misconceptions regarding the value of the electroencephalogram as a measure of a child's intellectual capacity are not only widespread among parents but also among teachers, social workers, nurses, and a number of other professionals who deal with children suffering from various kinds of physical and mental handicaps or from learning problems.

What other diagnostic tests can be performed on a child with seizures and when are these tests indicated?

I said earlier that the routine diagnostic investigation of a child with seizures includes a few blood and urine tests, skull x-rays, and an electroencephalogram. Indications for additional diagnostic studies depend on the results of these tests and especially on the medical history and on the results of the physical examination of the child. If the examination shows abnormal findings, the physician may decide to perform additional diagnostic tests. Among these we should mention the brain scan, the echoencephalogram, the ventriculogram, the pneumoencephalogram and the brain angiogram.

The brain scan involves the injection of a very small amount of radioactive material into the vein of an arm. One-half to one hour after its injection the material reaches its maximal concentration in the brain. At this time, special x-rays of the skull are taken and areas of abnormal concentration (uptake) of the radioactive material within the brain are looked for. Lesions such as brain tumors, congenitally malformed cerebral blood vessels, or bleeding inside the skull can show discrete areas of increased uptake of the radioactive material on the x-ray.

In the echoencephalogram an ultrasound beam is sent from

one side of the skull to the other. As the ultrasound beam travels through the brain it sends an echo each time it hits an area of different density. This echo, which is similar to a radar signal, can be recorded on Polaroid film. The procedure is entirely safe, painless, and can be performed on an outpatient basis. The echoencephalogram, then, essentially provides information regarding the position of certain brain structures and their possible displacement from their usual locations by lesions such as brain tumors, abscesses, or bleeding.

The ventriculogram and the pneumoencephalogram are special forms of x-rays of the skull taken after a certain amount of spinal fluid has been removed and replaced by air. When the cavities (ventricles) that are normally present in the center of the brain are filled with air, they become visible in x-rays of the skull taken with the head in different positions. In this way, physicians are able to assess the exact configuration and position of the ventricles as well as any possible displacement of them caused by lesions such as tumor, or by other lesions which produce pressure on the brain.

The brain angiogram consists of the injection of a special dye into a large artery in the neck with the purpose of visualizing the blood vessels (arteries and veins) inside the brain. In children, a simpler and safer procedure is to insert a catheter in a large artery of the groin and pass it all the way up into one of the large vessels at the base of the neck. When the catheter is in the latter position, dye is injected. As the dye travels through the vessels of the brain, serial x-rays of the skull are taken to demonstrate their patency and location.

The previously mentioned diagnostic tests are performed in children with seizures only when there are more or less clear-cut indications for them. The brain scan and the echoencephalogram are entirely safe tests which can be performed on an outpatient basis. The ventriculogram, pneumoencephalogram, and angiogram need to be done while the patient is hospitalized; all three of them carry a small risk. Unless the cause of epilepsy is a lesion, such as a brain tumor, or a group of congenitally malformed cerebral blood vessels (arteriovenous malformation), these tests rarely provide an answer as to the cause of a child's recurrent seizures. Therefore, unless clearly indicated, tests such as the ventriculogram, pneumoencephalogram, or angiogram have a limited place in the diagnosis of epilepsy. They are not entirely safe. They are not inexpensive, either.

You said that a brain scan involves the injection of radioactive material. Isn't that dangerous?

No, it is not. The amount of radioactivity produced by the injected material is less than the amount of radioactivity produced by a chest x-ray.

5. How Is Epilepsy Treated?

Who takes care of children with seizures?

Until approximately fifteen years ago the great majority of children with epilepsy were treated by pediatricians, family physicians, neurosurgeons, or adult neurologists. In more recent years, and as a result of the ever-increasing number of medical specialists, a new breed of child physician has become primarily concerned with the diagnosis and management of diseases of the nervous system of infants and children. He or she is called a pediatric neurologist, and as the name implies it is a rather strange cross between a pediatrician and a neurologist. Thus far, however, the number of practicing pediatric neurologists in this country is too small to take care of all children with seizures, let alone evaluate, manage, and follow up all children with disorders affecting the nervous system. Therefore, today as ten years ago, the great majority of epileptic children are diagnosed, treated, and followed up by pediatricians or family physicians. Parents should rest assured that there is nothing wrong with this policy. In this respect we should point out that present medical-school curriculums and postgraduate training of pediatricians and family physicians include fairly comprehensive teaching and experience in the diagnosis and treatment of seizures in children as well as adults.

Should every child with seizures be initially examined or subsequently followed up by a neurologist?

In selected cases, yes. As a routine policy, no. I believe that in the great majority of instances this is neither necessary nor feasible. If we consider that there are approximately two million children with epilepsy in the United States and only about four thousand neurologists, of whom two hundred and fifty have received specialized training in the treatment of neurologic problems of infancy and childhood, it becomes quite clear that such a small group of physicians cannot possibly take care of such a large number of children.

Is this a serious drawback in the management of children with seizures?

Not at all. As noted above, the great majority of epileptic children can be adequately diagnosed and properly treated by pediatricians or family physicians. The diagnosis and treatment of seizures is neither an esoteric matter nor does it require very highly specialized medical training. You may be sure that, if a child's seizures are difficult to control, or if he has other neurological problems, your pediatrician or family physician will refer your child for consultation to a neurologist. Because of the small number of neurologists, they are usually available for consultation in only fairly large cities.

Parents of children with seizures should know that a number of states have special clinics for the diagnosis and treatment of children with epilepsy. Many of these clinics are partially supported either by state funds or by funds from the Children's Bureau of the Department of Health, Education, and Welfare. Also many large hospitals and medical centers, especially those associated with medical schools, have seizure clinics for both children and adults. If parents are not familiar with the facilities available in a particular state, the

Epilepsy Foundation of America,* a nonprofit organization, can supply the names of available clinics in a particular vicinity, or the names of physicians especially interested in the care of children with epilepsy.

How often is it possible to get rid of the cause of seizures?

Not very often. Unfortunately the elimination of the cause of seizures can be accomplished only in a very small percentage of children with epilepsy. Treatable conditions that may cause recurrent seizures, such as hypoglycemia (low blood glucose), hypocalcemia (low blood calcium), or intoxications are curable but, as we have seen, they represent only a very small percentage of children with seizures.

What can be done, then, for the millions of children who do not have a curable condition?

As soon as a diagnosis of epileptic seizures is made, all these children should receive medications on a continuous, daily basis to prevent the occurrence of further seizures. This can be done with one or more of several excellent anticonvulsant drugs presently available for the treatment of the several different types of seizures.

Can treatment with anticonvulsant drugs also prevent the recurrence of febrile seizures?

At the present time nobody seems to have a precise answer for this question. The efficacy of daily anticonvulsant treatment in the prevention of febrile seizures is still a matter of controversy among specialists in epilepsy and child neurology. Some physicians feel that a child with febrile seizures of short duration, who has a normal electroencephalogram seven days after recovery from fever, and who does not show per-

* Epilepsy Foundation of America, 1419 H Street, N.W., Washington, D.C. 20005.

manent neurologic signs or some evidence of a structural brain lesion, should receive medications to lower fever plus anticonvulsant drugs *only* at the time of subsequent febrile illnesses. On the other hand, other physicians believe that all children with febrile seizures should be treated with continuous, daily anticonvulsant therapy until they reach the age of five or six years; the rationale for this rather drastic policy being that, in our present state of knowledge, it is extremely difficult, if not impossible, to differentiate a simple febrile seizure from an epileptic attack brought on by fever. An additional argument offered by the proponents of daily, prolonged anticonvulsant treatment is that approximately 10 to 20 percent of children who have febrile seizures will, at a later age, have seizures in the absence of fever, and will then have to be regarded and treated as epileptics. Physicians who treat infants and young children with febrile seizures thus hope that daily treatment with anticonvulsant medication until the age of five years will not only prevent further recurrence of febrile seizures but will also prevent the occurrence of nonfebrile seizures in that 10 to 20 percent of youngsters who statistically can be expected to develop seizures in the absence of fever.

Who is right?

I wish I knew for certain. I have said before that it is not easy for physicians to differentiate between a simple, benign febrile seizure and a seizure precipitated by fever in a young child who happens to be an epileptic. My personal policy, therefore, is dictated exclusively by pragmatic considerations, and I wouldn't be surprised if sooner rather than later I am proved to be utterly wrong. Nevertheless, since I have no way of knowing with certainty which child will fall into that 10 to 20 percent mentioned above, my own decision is to treat all children with febrile seizures with daily, continuous anticonvulsant drugs, almost always phenobarbital, while being perfectly aware that by doing so I may be treating unnecessarily 80 to 90 percent of children with febrile seizures.

Recent reports indicate that continuous, daily treatment with *adequate* amounts of phenobarbital is of value in preventing the recurrence of febrile seizures, and that what physicians have called in the past benign febrile seizures may not be benign after all. Up to now physicians have been divided into two irreconcilable groups in regard to the treatment of febrile seizures. It may well be that the pendulum will swing in the near future toward those who recommend continuous anticonvulsant therapy for all children with febrile seizures.

How do anticonvulsant medicines work?

The exact mechanism of action of anticonvulsant drugs remains largely unknown. This shouldn't come as a surprise to anybody. The same is true of other relatively simple drugs, like aspirin, which have been around for a much longer time. The only thing physicians know for certain is that anticonvulsant drugs increase the seizure threshold (brain resistance to seizures) for a particular type of spell. For example, Dilantin, one of the most useful and widely used drugs in the treatment of epilepsy, raises four times the seizure threshold of cats to convulsions produced by electric shock. To put it in other words, when cats are given a certain amount of Dilantin, convulsions occur only if the intensity of the electric shock is four times stronger than the amount of electricity needed to produce the same type of convulsion when the animal has not received the drug.

Some antiepileptic drugs appear to act directly on the discharging brain cells and dampen the abnormal electrical discharges. Others seem to prevent the spreading of the electrical disturbances from their site of origin to neighboring nerve cells and in this way stop the electrical buildup which eventually leads to a seizure.

Which is the best drug for the treatment of seizures?

None. There is no such thing as the single best drug for the treatment of epileptic seizures. An excellent drug for the prevention of one type of seizure may be totally ineffective in the prevention of another type of seizure. Furthermore, sometimes a useful drug in the treatment of one type of seizure may make more severe or increase the number of spells of another type. Dilantin, for example, an excellent drug for the treatment of grand mal and psychomotor seizures, may increase the frequency of petit mal attacks, and Tridione, a useful drug in the treatment of petit mal, may precipitate a first grand mal attack or increase their frequency if they have already occurred.

How effective are drugs in the treatment of seizures?

With the anticonvulsants currently available in the market, seizures can be brought under complete control in about 70 percent of cases. In an additional 20 percent there is a considerable decrease in the frequency or in the severity of seizures or both; and in 10 percent there is either no improvement whatever, or the seizures get worse.

At present physicians have at their disposal a large number of excellent drugs for the prevention of epileptic seizures. There can be no doubt that some of these drugs are more effective than others. It should be pointed out, however, that when we say that one drug is better than another, what we really mean is that over the years that particular drug has been found to be more effective in preventing spells in a large number of patients with a certain type of seizure. Occasionally, a second-choice anticonvulsant may stop seizures in a given child when one or more of the first-choice drugs have failed to do so.

Is it possible for a physician to tell parents in advance whether medication will control their child's seizures?

Since the great majority of patients with epilepsy can be adequately controlled with anticonvulsant drugs, many physicians tend to be on the optimistic side and will answer this question with an unqualified "yes." Actually, all one can do is to evaluate each individual child in regard to a number of variables, among them the possible cause of the seizures, their type, their frequency and severity, and the kind of changes which may be present in the electroencephalogram. When all these factors are put together, the physician may, at best, give an educated estimate as to the chances for control based either on his personal or somebody else's experience.

When patients with different types of seizures are lumped together, we arrive at the figures given above: 70 percent for complete control and an additional 20 percent who will experience either a decrease in the severity of the seizures or a decrease in their frequency. When one considers the probabilities of success in relation to the different types of seizures the picture changes quite a bit. Some seizures are easy to control; others are not. It is almost ironic that, with the exception of petit mal, all other forms of seizures referred to as minor are in most cases difficult to bring under control for any prolonged period of time. Children with minor motor seizures (myoclonic and akinetic) usually respond initially very well to treatment, but, for some reason, sooner or later the seizures have a tendency to break through. On the other hand, grand mal, the most common and also the most dramatic form of epilepsy, is probably the easiest one to bring under complete control.

The degree of success in the treatment of any type of seizure depends primarily on a proper diagnosis. Since the only way of giving seizures their accurate name is by taking a detailed history of the attacks, it is necessary to re-emphasize that it is of paramount importance to elicit an accurate and complete history of the attacks. This enables the physician to give the proper name to the type of seizure a child is having in the great majority of cases and thus to prescribe the medication most likely to stop them. We can see, then, how parents who are good observers and better historians can be of great help to the physician.

For how long have drugs been used in the treatment of seizures?

Physicians have been using drugs in one form or another in the treatment of epileptic seizures for more than two thousand years. In ancient Greece physicians often resorted to a combination of substances derived from animal organs, and to magic in the form of amulets, and to special rituals to counteract the supernatural factors believed to be involved in the causation of seizures.

During the Middle Ages the same old approaches to treatment continued to be generally used. In addition, physicians began to rely heavily on charms and exorcisms. New methods of treatment such as mistletoe potion and castration were introduced in mentally ill patients whose epileptic attacks were believed to be precipitated by masturbation. For hundreds of years mistletoe potion remained a very popular medicine for the treatment of seizures. The reason for its use was the belief that, because of the strong attachment of mistletoe to the branches of the oak tree, a potion made from it had to be effective against the "falling sickness."

Until the middle of the nineteenth century there was no truly effective drug for the treatment of epilepsy. In 1853 Sir Charles Locock in England first reported on the beneficial effect of bromide salts in a group of patients with seizures who were receiving this medication for totally unrelated purposes. Thus, almost by accident bromide salts became the first effective drug in the treatment of epilepsy. The amount of bromide needed to control certain types of seizures, however, often produced marked mental dullness and disfiguring skin eruptions. The widespread use of bromide salts was probably a factor which reinforced in the mind of the general public the erroneous idea that epilepsy was a condition leading to progressive mental deterioration and insanity.

The modern era of drug therapy of epilepsy began in 1912 when Dr. Alfred Hauptman in Germany introduced phenobarbital as the drug of choice in the treatment of seizures. Phenobarbital, still today one of the best and most widely used anticonvulsant drugs, remained for all practical purposes the only effective form of therapy until 1938, when dyphenylhydantoin (Dilantin), another extremely useful drug, was introduced. In contrast to phenobarbital, Dilantin was found to have potent anticonvulsant properties without producing sedation or hypnotic effects. Since 1938 a number of other drugs also highly effective in the treatment of different types of seizures have become available. Among these, we should mention Mysoline, Zarontin, Tridione, Paradione, Celontin, Milontin, and Valium.

How do physicians know how much medicine a child is supposed to take?

The amount of daily drug needed to control seizures as well as the maximal amount of it that a child can tolerate is by now fairly well standardized. This amount or dosage depends basically on two factors: the weight and the age of the child. Infants and young children appear to eliminate anticonvulsants from the body much faster than adults. In general, therefore, they need a larger amount of drug in relation to their body weight than grownups.

How do physicians know that a child is actually getting the amount of drug he needs?

The ideal amount of any anticonvulsant drug is that which controls seizures without producing adverse effects such as drowsiness, sleepiness, or unsteadiness of gait, which will obviously interfere with the child's well-being. The achievement of this ideal amount of medication, however, may need frequent adjustments in the daily dosage of one or more drugs, and also very often a great deal of patience on the part of both parents and physicians.

What can be done if one drug does not control seizures?

In most cases, if a drug has been properly chosen according to a particular type of seizure, it will almost always be of some benefit. Even though the child may continue to have seizures, they will be less severe or less frequent. As long as a drug is effective, its dosage can be increased until seizures are brought completely under control or until the child develops undesirable side effects. If the first drug does not completely stop seizures at high dosages, a second drug can be given in addition to the first one, and then again increased in dosage until seizures are under control or until side effects appear. In an occasional case three or more drugs may have to be given to gain complete control of seizures. It cannot be stressed enough that *any increase in the dosage of one medication or the addition of new ones should be made only by the physician treating the child.* Only he is in a position to decide when an increase in dosage is still indicated and safe, or that the time has come when it will be necessary to introduce a new drug.

What if the child has two different types of seizures?

In the great majority of cases if a child has more than one type of seizure, a single drug will probably prove unsuccessful in controlling seizures. Combined drug therapy, with two or more different drugs, is usually required to control patients with more than one type of attack.

How safe are drugs used in the treatment of seizures?

No drug used in the treatment of any disease has yet proved to be 100 percent safe. In the case of drugs used in the treatment of seizures, the problem of safety is, at least theoretically, compounded by the fact that in most cases they have to be given for prolonged periods of time, usually at least three or more years. Fortunately some of the most effective and commonly used drugs in the treatment of epilepsy are much safer than aspirin. Others are not. At any rate, although mild side effects are fairly common, serious complications are rare and can be detected early enough if parents make it a custom to report to their physician any unusual and persistent symptoms. Physicians in turn perform periodic blood, urine, or liver tests when the prescribed drug is known to be potentially toxic for the blood-forming organs, the kidneys, or the liver. As noted above, the majority of commonly-used drugs in the treatment of epilepsy are as safe as any other drug in use at the present time. Some of the commonly used anticonvulsants are actually safer than most drugs used in the treatment of a number of chronic illnesses affecting other organs.

The "ideal" drug for the treatment of any condition should meet at least three requirements: it should be effective in 100 percent of the patients in whom it is used; it should be totally free of unpleasant side effects or serious complications; and it should be cheap. Phenobarbital, one of the most effective and commonly used drugs in the treatment of seizures, is as close to being an ideal drug as any that we know.

How soon after the beginning of treatment can one expect a decrease in the number or complete control of seizures?

It is not always possible to predict when. Parents should not get discouraged if the number of seizures a child is having remains unchanged for a few days up to one or two weeks after the beginning of treatment. It has been estimated that effective concentrations of anticonvulsants in the blood and the brain are usually not reached until about one to two weeks after the beginning of treatment. Parents ought to remember also that it is always possible that even when adequate blood concentrations of a drug are achieved the seizures may still not be completely controlled.

Nowadays when physicians have at their disposal so many excellent drugs it is not difficult to understand why parents and patients alike expect immediate and long-lasting results from the use of just about any medicine. This attitude is to be discouraged in parents of children with epilepsy. Although on a purely statistical basis the great majority of them will improve on drug treatment, parents should be fully aware that the road to success sometimes may be full of difficulties and frustrations.

For how long should an epileptic child receive daily medication to prevent seizures?

At the present time the consensus among specialists in epilepsy and child neurology is that any child with a chronic seizure disorder should receive continuous, daily anticonvulsant treatment for at least three years after the last seizure. The dosage is then usually tapered off over a period of nine to twelve months and finally discontinued altogether. Since the amount of anticonvulsant drug prescribed to children with epilepsy depends primarily on body weight, as long as a child has been free of seizures for a prolonged period of time, a spontaneous tapering-off of the medication can be expected to occur as he gains in weight. If a very large amount of anticonvulsant or several drugs has been needed to gain control of seizures, the treating physician may deem it necessary to prolong this tapering-off period for more than twelve months.

Parents should never forget that the decision to taper off or discontinue an anticonvulsant drug should be made only by a physician. We often see parents who, because their child has not had a seizure for six or twelve months, discontinue anticonvulsants either because they have decided on their own that he no longer needs them, or worse, just to see what will happen. Parents should realize that there is more involved in the decision to discontinue anticonvulsant drugs than just a certain seizure-free period of three or more years. Other factors, such as the probable cause of a child's seizures, and the presence or absence of abnormalities in the electroencephalogram, also need to be taken into consideration. It is obvious, then, that parents should have no part in this decision-making process. Only the treating physician, after several factors are taken into consideration, is in a position to make such a delicate decision.

Most drugs used in the treatment of seizures are available in tablet or in suspension (liquid) form. What are the advantages or disadvantages of tablets versus suspensions?

On first thought there would seem to be only one difference: tablets are solid and suspensions are liquid. But there is probably much more to it than just a difference in physical properties. In contrast to popular belief, I am convinced that in most cases the advantages of tablets over suspensions are many. For one thing, tablets do not have to be shaken. This is not meant to be a joke. If parents forget to shake the bottle with the suspension, they may be giving the child too little of the medicine today and too much tomorrow. If they consistently forget to do this, it is more than likely that the child will receive very little, if any, drug during an entire week and intoxicating amounts of it during the next one; the obvious result being that adequate blood levels of the drug will not be constantly maintained.

Liquid preparations often have to be given either in calibrated droppers or in calibrated teaspoons. We are all well aware that household teaspoons vary greatly in size; therefore, they cannot be relied upon if one attempts to measure accurately a certain amount of drug from a suspension which contains a fairly large amount of medicine per teaspoon. If by any chance a household teaspoon is used, the administration of one-half teaspoon becomes for all practical purposes some sort of a guessing game rather than an accurate determination. If a young child should spit up a portion of the suspension, it may be difficult, if not impossible, to estimate accurately the amount needed to replace it. This again may result in the administration of too little or too much anticonvulsant. Last but not least, all suspension preparations of anticonvulsants are several times more expensive than tablets. This is by no means an unimportant consideration when a child has to take medications for several years.

Is it not easier to give a liquid medicine to infants or young children rather than tablets?

No, it is not. It would seem that the answer to this question has to be a resounding "yes." We are convinced, however, that in the great majority of cases this is simply not true. First of all, I would like to support this statement by saying that I have never had any problems prescribing tablets to infants or young children as long as they were able to swallow. It is really not as difficult to give tablets to infants or young children as many parents seem to believe. The tablet, or a portion of it (most are scored), can be crushed and given mixed with one teaspoon of apple or banana sauce. Since many of the tablets are either tasteless or are flavored, the chances that the child will spit up a portion of it are very small. Some of the liquid preparations, on the other hand, are either not very tasty or because of their high alcohol content are downright unpalatable. Another practical disadvantage of liquid preparations is that they have to be prescribed in ten- or twelve-ounce bottles. The result of this is that parents end up making very frequent trips to the pharmacy. If this doesn't sound to you like too much of a nuisance, remember that it will go on for at least three years.

Do all anticonvulsant drugs come in suspension as well as in tablets and capsule forms?

No. But many of them do. The most notable exception in this respect was, until a few months ago, Zarontin, probably the most effective drug in the treatment of petit mal, which since its introduction in the market was available only as a liquid-filled capsule measuring three quarters of an inch.

Isn't this a rather large capsule for a young child to swallow? Are some children unable to take it?

A capsule of this size is definitely a very large one to swallow—and not only for young children, but for just about anybody. It is not at all surprising then that a fairly large number of young children who are prescribed this drug have difficulties in swallowing it.

What can be done if a child is unable or refuses to swallow a capsule this large and there is no other way to give the medication?

If this is the case, there are only two alternatives left. One is to make a hole in the capsule with a pin and squeeze the liquid content directly into the child's mouth. The second is to give it diluted in one-half or one ounce of sweet juice or milk. Either way is not very tasty. About a pint of very sweet juice is needed to counteract the unpleasant taste of the liquid content of the capsule. In our experience a less barbaric and much more successful method is to freeze the capsules and cut each one in two or three pieces at the time of administration.

As mentioned above, Zarontin has also become available

in a suspension form. In our opinion, this does not alter our belief that the advantages of capsules and tablets over suspensions are many. If your physician has prescribed Zarontin in capsule form, and your child has difficulty swallowing the capsule, you can follow the previously mentioned advice.

Can the same procedure be followed with other medications which are only available in capsule form?

No, the content of the overwhelming majority of medications manufactured in capsule form is powder and not liquid. And powder does not freeze easily, at least not in *your* freezer.

Isn't phenobarbital a barbiturate and therefore a potentially habit-forming drug?

Yes, it is. However, we must say that in our experience as well as that of hundreds of pediatricians and neurologists who have treated thousands of children with epilepsy for more than sixty years, addiction or dependency has not been a problem in children with epilepsy who have received the drug daily for several years. The only reason for this lack of dependency or addiction to phenobarbital or to other chemically related drugs is that phenobarbital, unlike other drugs such as morphine or heroin, is not a habit-forming drug. The same is not true, however, of other barbiturates such as Seconal or Nembutal (sleeping pills), which frequently cause dependency or addiction, especially when taken under no medical supervision by emotionally disturbed individuals.

Are there any other potentially habit-forming drugs among the many used in the treatment of epilepsy?

Several other medications used in the treatment of epilepsy are very closely related to phenobarbital from the standpoint of their chemical structure. They can also then be considered, at least from a theoretical standpoint, to fall into the category of potentially habit-forming drugs. But, as has been the case with phenobarbital, none of them have caused drug dependency or addiction in the millions of children treated for epilepsy for as long as five, ten, or more years. At present the great majority of drugs used in the treatment of epilepsy are not even potentially habit-forming.

Will treatment with phenobarbital, a well-known sedative, make the child dopy or interfere with his ability to learn?

Most unlikely. For some unknown reason children appear to be somewhat immune to the sedative effect of phenobarbital. At the dosages used in the treatment of seizures very few children experience undesirable side effects. Some children, especially older ones, may become drowsy or experience excessive somnolence during the first few weeks of treatment with phenobarbital. Subsequently most of them, however, are able to overcome this unpleasant side effect and are able to tolerate the same or larger amounts of the drug without experiencing undesirable side effects. An occasional child, however, will not "outgrow" these undesirable manifestations and will continue to be drowsy or somnolent. If phenobarbital has been effective in controlling the child's seizures, the physician may elect not to switch him to another anticonvulsant, but instead prescribe a small amount of another medication to counteract the sedative effect.

Experience with thousands of epileptic children who have taken phenobarbital or related drugs for several years have shown that if the child does not become somnolent, or drowsy, the prolonged administration of any of these drugs does not interfere with the child's ability to learn. For unknown reasons a large number of children who are prescribed phenobarbital, especially those who are mentally slow or who are hyperactive, do not become drowsy but instead experience what has been called "paradoxical reaction." A paradoxical reaction is said to occur when the administration of a certain drug produces exactly the opposite of its expected effect. In the case of phenobarbital, instead of the usual sedative effect produced by the drug, many children will become hyperactive, restless, jittery, or have difficulty falling asleep. It should be made clear that the antiepileptic effect of phenobarbital has no relation whatever to its sedative effect or its paradoxical effect. Thus, even though a child may experience a paradoxical reaction to the administration of phenobarbital it doesn't follow that the drug will also have a paradoxical or no effect at all on his seizures.

What can be done if a child should develop a paradoxical reaction to phenobarbital?

If a paradoxical reaction should occur, the physician is left with several alternatives. To a great extent these alternatives depend on the severity of the reaction. If this is mild, he may choose to wait for a reasonable period of time and see what happens. If the reaction is severe, to the point that the child may become unmanageable or difficult to live with, he may decide to replace phenobarbital with another anticonvulsant. In general, a switch to another anticonvulsant is not much of a problem since there are several other drugs in the market also effective in the treatment of the type of seizures for which phenobarbital is usually prescribed.

If a child gets used to the sedative effect of phenobarbital, will he also get used to or outgrow the antiepileptic effect of the drug?

It would seem only logical to think that both actions (sedative and antiepileptic) should go hand in hand. Fortunately this is not so. Although most children who exhibit a mild to moderate degree of drowsiness at the beginning of treatment will outgrow this unpleasant side effect, usually within a period of two to three weeks after the beginning of treatment, the antiepileptic efficacy of the drug remains unchanged.

Why, then, don't physicians start treatment with another drug which they know will not produce somnolence or drowsiness?

They often do. Remember that different types of seizures may require different kinds of anticonvulsants. And many of them produce neither drowsiness nor somnolence. We have already mentioned that phenobarbital is very close to being an ideal drug (effective, relatively free of side effects, and cheap). Although it is true that there are other drugs which are as effective as phenobarbital in the treatment of certain types of seizures and which do not cause drowsiness at the usual dosages, they are also less safe and much more expensive. When some of them are prescribed, physicians have to perform periodic blood or other tests to detect and prevent at an early stage the development of anemia, or other problems which may affect the blood-forming tissues or other organs. A word of reassurance is in order. The number of children who develop serious complications as a result of prolonged administration of anticonvulsants is, indeed, extremely small when compared with the hundreds of thousands of patients who take these medications on a daily basis for many years and never experience any difficulties.

What are some of the other possible complications of anticonvulsant treatment?

With two or three exceptions all antiepileptic drugs may produce toxic effects in organs such as the liver, the kidneys, or the blood-forming organs. It must be re-emphasized, however, that the number of patients who develop such complications from the use of these drugs is extremely small. If complications are going to occur, they will usually develop during the first few months after the beginning of treatment. For this reason physicians perform the appropriate laboratory tests at fairly frequent intervals during the first few months of treatment and later on usually every three to four months, or at more frequent intervals, according to the type and number of drugs a child is taking.

What can be done if a child develops one of these complications?

Some of the mild side effects produced by treatment with anticonvulsants can be managed simply by decreasing the daily amount of the drug. More severe reactions, however, may require the withdrawal of the drug and its replacement by another anticonvulsant. In the overwhelming majority of children in whom a serious complication arises, withdrawal of the drug will bring a halt to the problem. Permanent damage to the blood-forming organs, liver, or kidneys is a distinctly rare occurrence. Whenever a child who is taking anticonvulsant drugs develops any side effects, his parents should get in touch with their physician. He is the only one who can evaluate the situation and make a decision as to whether the drug should be withdrawn temporarily, indefinitely, or its daily dosage decreased.

Is overdosage with anticonvulsants a rare occurrence?

Not at all. As a matter of fact it is much more common than parents think it possible.

Johnny just couldn't have taken an overdose. He is only three years old, and we always make sure to keep the bottle of medicine out of his reach in a kitchen (or bathroom) cabinet.

There are only two ways by which a child can get an overdose. He may either accidentally be given one or he may accidentally chew or swallow a large number of tablets or a large amount of suspension on his own. How can parents give the child an overdose? For one thing, it is always possible that parents, knowingly or unknowingly, may disregard their physicians' instructions. In our experience, however, this situation is a rare occurrence. On the other hand, an excessive administration of anticonvulsants is not very uncommon when drugs are given in suspension form.

How can this happen?

There is more than one possibility. By mistake, parents may give the drug in teaspoons instead of cc.s (metric measure of volume used by physicians and equivalent to one-fifth of a teaspoon). When the prescribed suspension of a drug comes in two different concentrations, the pharmacist may inadvertently dispense a suspension which may be four or five times stronger than that prescribed by the physician. I must admit that pharmacists rarely make this type of mistake. They can, though. I have seen it happen at least three times in the last couple of years. In pediatric practice the most common error in this respect occurs with Dilantin, which comes in two suspensions of very different concentrations: a red suspension which contains thirty milligrams per teaspoon and a creamy-white suspension which contains one hundred and twenty-five milligrams per teaspoon. Thus far we have seen so many children who became moderately intoxicated when Dilantin was given in suspension form that we have made it a custom whenever we prescribe it to warn parents that they should make sure the pharmacist always refills the suspension of the same color. Hoping of course that the suspension of the correct color was dispensed the first time!

How could my three-year-old child have taken an overdose? We have already told you how careful we are in keeping medicines in a place where he cannot possibly reach them.

It is surprising to what extent parents can underestimate the ability of toddlers to open bottles, or the ingenuity of young children at getting into what appears to be an inaccessible kitchen or bathroom cabinet. Because the child with epilepsy needs to take anticonvulsants for a prolonged period of time, they are usually dispensed in one hundred or two hundred tablets or capsules at a time. Thus, if accidental ingestion of tablets or capsules is suspected, more often than not it is extremely difficult, if not impossible, to tell just by looking at the bottle whether the child might have taken an extra five, ten, or twenty tablets.

What should parents do if a child accidentally ingests a large number of tablets or capsules or swallows a large amount of suspension?

Get in touch with your physician immediately. Emptying and washing out of the stomach can be done within two hours following ingestion of the drug in an attempt to get rid of some of the ingested drug. Because symptoms of intoxication usually do not appear until a few hours after the child has taken an overdose, this method of treatment is not always feasible. Two hours after ingestion, the drug has either been absorbed in the stomach or traveled down the gut.

What are the symptoms of an overdose?

Intoxication with any anticonvulsant is almost always manifested by somnolence, drowsiness, severe unsteadiness of gait, stupor, and finally a state of deep sleep (coma) from which the child cannot be aroused. If the ingested amount is large enough, respiratory arrest or circulatory collapse may ensue. It is mandatory then that any child who has ingested an overdose be immediately examined by a physician.

An effort should be made by both parents and physician to determine the amount of drug ingested. Since the great majority of epileptic children take anticonvulsant drugs on a regular schedule (usually two to four times daily), a fairly accurate estimate of the amount ingested can be made by counting the number of tablets that should be left in the bottle according to the date in which the prescription was filled and the number dispensed by the pharmacist. A similar method of calculation can be used if the drug was ingested in suspension form. If there are doubts regarding the possibility of overdose, the easiest and safest way to find out whether a few tablets or capsules may be missing from the bottle is to call the pharmacist and ask him for the number of them dispensed in the original prescription and the date on which this was filled. We have found this to be the most expedient and reliable way of finding out in a short period of time the exact number of tablets or capsules which may be missing from the bottle. Once the amount of anticonvulsant drug ingested can be established, the physician is in a position to decide whether the patient can be returned to his home, kept in the hospital for a period of observation, or hospitalized for immediate treatment.

Unfortunately there is no specific antidote for intoxication with anticonvulsant drugs. Nevertheless, if the patient is severely intoxicated, he will need supportive treatment for any respiratory or circulatory problems which might develop while his body slowly gets rid of the drug. In cases of severe intoxications with certain anticonvulsants, the physician can accelerate the elimination of the drug from the body by one of several techniques, known as peritoneal dialysis, hemodialysis, or exchange transfusion.

Is there any other way to find out the amount of medicine a child may have accidentally taken?

Yes. In recent years laboratory methods to measure the amount of anticonvulsant present in the blood have become available. At present, however, few hospitals in the country have the necessary facilities to do this type of determination.

It should be re-emphasized that the accidental ingestion of an overdose of anticonvulsants by young children is not a very unusual occurrence. Because of this, if a child is receiving daily anticonvulsant drugs and develops unusual symptoms which cannot be readily explained by one of the common diseases of childhood, he should be considered to have received an overdose until it has been proven otherwise. Symptoms that parents ought to watch for are unexplained changes in the level of consciousness, such as excessive somnolence or drowsiness, and sudden changes in coordination and gait. If in doubt, always call your physician.

Dilantin, one of the most effective anticonvulsant drugs, often produces marked swelling of the gums. Is there anything that can be done to prevent or minimize this problem?

Yes. And it all boils down to keeping the teeth clean. First, let us mention that swelling or hypertrophy of the gums is not a serious complication of Dilantin therapy and is seldom a compelling reason for withdrawal of the drug, especially if it has proved effective in controlling the child's seizures. Gum hypertrophy rarely occurs in adults but is observed in approximately 40 percent of children who take Dilantin for a prolonged period of time. The upper gums are almost always more affected than the lower gums. This cosmetic side effect is not related to the amount of drug taken; it is probably due to individual susceptibility to the drug. There can be little doubt, however, that the accumulation of debris and plaque on the teeth and between the teeth and gums also plays a significant role in the development of gum hypertrophy. This is supported by the fact that meticulous oral hygiene seems to prevent it almost completely. The best way to maintain healthy teeth and gums is by cleaning the gingival sulcus (where the gums meet the teeth) with a soft-bristle brush, performing a circular scrubbing motion, and by the daily use of dental floss to remove plaque and debris from the upper portion of the spaces between the teeth which are left untouched by the toothbrush. Parents should carry out this "ordeal," or supervise the child, once daily until he has learned to perform it satisfactorily.

Once gum hypertrophy has developed not even the most vigorous massage of the gums will be of any benefit in decreasing the amount of swelling. In some instances it is necessary that the dentist remove surgically excessive amounts of gum tissue. In some children orthodontic treatment is necessary to correct displacement of teeth caused by gum hypertrophy.

Can swollen gums due to Dilantin therapy become a permanent problem?

No. The gums remain swollen only as long as the child is taking Dilantin. They will always return to their normal size following withdrawal of the drug. This may take anywhere from three to twelve months.

My six-year-old daughter had two convulsions six months ago during a two-week period. She has been taking Dilantin for about five months. For the past three months we have noticed she is growing long dark hair on her legs, arm, back, and fuzzy stuff over the sides of her jaws. Is this due to the medicine? And if so what can be done about it?

Excessive hair growth on parts of the body on which it is cosmetically undesirable, especially in a little girl, is not an uncommon complication of Dilantin therapy; it occurs in about 5 percent of people taking Dilantin for a prolonged period of time. The undesirable aspect of excessive hair growth resulting from Dilantin therapy is that, in contrast to gum swelling, once developed, it doesn't go away. Discuss the problem with your physician. The sooner you do this the better. He may decide to switch her to another anticonvulsant drug. If Dilantin is indispensable for satisfactory control of her seizures, there may not be an alternative other than to put up with it. If Dilantin is dispensable, a switch to another anticonvulsant may be worth trying. The psychological and emotional trauma of a heavy mustache or hairy legs can certainly be, in the long run, a much more serious problem than seizures, especially if the child is a female.

Why do you mention so many side effects of phenobarbital and Dilantin therapy? Previously you said that at present several excellent anticonvulsants are available for the treatment of seizures.

Neither propaganda nor personal interest. I own no stocks in any pharmaceutical company. The reason is only medical. Phenobarbital and Dilantin are by far the most widely used and effective drugs in the treatment of epilepsy in children as well as adults.

In Appendix 1, I have listed the most commonly used drugs in the treatment of seizures in infancy and childhood, the type of attacks for which they are most effective, their most important toxic effects, and the preparations available on the market.

If a child is taking more than one drug, can they be given at the same time of the day?

Yes. When given at the same time, none of the drugs presently used in the treatment of epilepsy appears to interfere with another one in regard to their absorption by the intestine. Occasionally, drugs used in the treatment of epilepsy may produce mild stomach irritation, especially when taken on an empty stomach. Therefore, it is not only convenient, but it may also be beneficial to the child if he receives two or more drugs at mealtimes or otherwise as indicated by the physician. If a particular drug produces stomach upset and has to be taken between meals, we recommend that it be taken with a glass of milk. In most instances this simple measure will eliminate the feeling of nausea or mild stomach discomfort that some children experience.

Do anticonvulsant drugs have to be given exactly at certain hours?

Not exactly at certain hours but at more or less regular intervals. For adequate control of any type of seizure, it is necessary that a fairly stable level of anticonvulsant be present at all times in the blood. This can be accomplished by dividing the total amount of drug which a child is supposed to take during a given day and giving it in two or more equal dosages at reasonably regular intervals. Some anticonvulsants remain in the body for a longer time and can be given in two divided daily dosages; others are eliminated more rapidly and have to be given at more frequent intervals. For example, the physician may choose to prescribe a drug in two divided doses, to be given at breakfast, and before going to bed. If a drug is prescribed in three daily doses, the noon dose is usually given in school at lunchtime or immediately after the child returns from school. This policy of giving anticonvulsant at one or more mealtimes and before going to bed is sound from a medical standpoint; blood levels of the drug are maintained within the desired levels even though the intervals between doses is not "exactly" the same. It is also convenient and practical; the chances that parents may forget to give the child his medication are certainly reduced if drugs are given at the time the child is sitting down to one or more of his meals and at bedtime.

In some cases a child may have seizures only at certain hours of the day or only during the night, and the prescribing physician may elect to give a larger amount of anticonvulsant a few hours prior to this time in an attempt to increase the amount of drug reaching the brain when it is most needed. Although there is no scientific proof that this is indeed accomplished, all of us at one time or another have made this type of recommendation. Deep down I have often been left with the uncomfortable feeling that by doing this I was appeasing myself rather than treating the patient. At any rate, only your physician is responsible for making decisions as to how the total amount of daily anticonvulsant is to be divided and the time of the day at which it should be taken.

A child with epilepsy is supposed to take his medicine "religiously" two or more times daily for a certain number of years. You have already mentioned that sudden withdrawal of anticonvulsants is dangerous: it may result in seizure recurrence after a prolonged seizure-free period or may even result in status epilepticus, which is a potentially dangerous situation. What can be done then if a child is for some reason unable to take or retain drugs by mouth?

Consult your physician. If your child has vomiting due to intestinal "flu" or other common diseases of childhood, your physician may prescribe a medicine to alleviate this symptom. If in spite of symptomatic treatment the child is still unable to retain drugs by mouth for a fairly prolonged period of time, the only alternative may be to give medications by intramuscular injection.

The risk of withdrawing medicines abruptly varies according to the type of seizures a child has and the drug he is receiving. If a child, for example, has petit mal and is receiving a drug such as Zarontin to prevent the occurrence of further spells, the chances that the withdrawal of this anticonvulsant will cause status epilepticus of grand mal type are practically nonexistent. He may have a recurrence of petit mal attacks, but he will not develop grand mal seizures *be-*

cause of withdrawal of Zarontin. On the other hand, if a child is receiving Dilantin, phenobarbital, or a related drug for the treatment of grand mal, psychomotor, or other type of seizures, there is always the possibility that sudden withdrawal of these medications may precipitate one or more grand mal seizures, even though the child may never have had one in the past.

In summary, the possibility of serious complications, such as status epilepticus, following sudden withdrawal of anti-convulsants depends not so much on the type of seizure a child has had in the past, but on the type of medicine he is taking. This is supported by the fact that a first grand mal seizure or even status epilepticus can occur after abrupt withdrawal of Dilantin or phenobarbital in people who have been taking these drugs for a prolonged period of time for conditions other than epilepsy.

Do you mean that phenobarbital and Dilantin are also used in the treatment of conditions other than epilepsy?

Yes, they are and have been used for a number of years. Phenobarbital, a drug synthetized at the beginning of this century, was initially made available to the medical profession as an excellent sedative. Only a few months after its introduction it was found that, in addition to being a sedative, phenobarbital also had outstanding anticonvulsant properties.

Dilantin, on the other hand, a drug which came into existence as an anticonvulsant as the result of a deliberate effort by a group of researchers to find an effective anticonvulsant without sedative properties, has ended up as one of the most versatile drugs used in medicine. In addition to its primary role as anticonvulsant, it is also used today in the treatment of migraine headaches, irregularities of heartbeat, trigeminal neuralgia, and a number of other conditions.

Is there any other treatment for epilepsy besides drugs?

Yes. It has been known for hundreds of years that fasting has a favorable effect on seizures. During the early part of this century, Dr. R. M. Wilder of the Mayo Clinic devised a special diet with which he attempted to reproduce the chemical changes which take place in the human body during starvation. While on this diet people accumulate in their bodies a large amount of substances called ketones. Because of this, the diet became known as the ketogenic diet. It consists essentially of the administration of a diet high in fat and very low in carbohydrates. The exact mechanism by which the ketogenic diet is effective in controlling some types of seizures remains unknown. It is generally accepted that its effect is due to a shift of the body metabolism toward acidosis (accumulation of an excessive amount of acid compounds in the blood and tissues). Since a large number of excellent drugs are nowadays available for the treatment of epilepsy, the ketogenic diet is used only in the occasional patient who does not respond to drug therapy. This is only one reason, however. There are several other drawbacks to its use. For one thing, if it is going to be effective, the patient has to adhere to it very strictly. Even minor dietary indiscretions, like eating two or three pieces of candy, may lower the amount of ketone substances present in the blood and throw the child off the state of ketosis. It goes without saying then that the diet must be rigorously controlled and that the child has to be closely supervised by his parents. In addition to the difficulties in meticulously preparing separate meals for the child, his urine has to be tested at least once a day to ensure that the desired chemical changes are indeed taking place and that they are more or less constantly maintained at the desired level.

Owing to the high content of fat and the small content of carbohydrates, most patients find the diet downright unpalatable. As a matter of fact very few adults or older children will strictly adhere to it for any prolonged period of time. Because of these limitations, experience has shown that the best candidates for this type of dietary management of epilepsy are preschool children between the ages of two and five years. As if this weren't enough, most physicians believe, and we agree on this, that it is usually necessary to hospitalize the child to start him on the diet. During this period of hospitalization, his mother can at the same time receive instructions from the dietician about the many details concerning the calculation and preparation of the diet. I am not fond of the ketogenic diet. I must admit, however, that I use it occasionally when everything else has failed to control a child's seizures. It is not only unpalatable, expensive, and difficult to prepare; it doesn't work in all cases either.

Can epilepsy be "cured" by surgery? It would seem only logical to go after the little scar or small portion of the brain from where seizures originate and take it out.

Yes, this can be done. Unfortunately the number of children who qualify as good candidates for surgical treatment is extremely small. There is unanimous agreement among physicians that surgical treatment of seizures is justified only when the patient fulfills the following criteria: (1) he has intractable and incapacitating seizures in spite of an adequate trial on anticonvulsant medications; (2) his electroencephalogram shows a well-localized epileptogenic area in a part of the brain which can be safely removed without producing serious motor or mental disabilities; and (3) an experienced surgical team is available to perform this type of surgery. At the present time, surgical treatment for epilepsy is done almost exclusively in patients with psychomotor seizures who have a well-defined epileptogenic focus in only one temporal lobe of the brain. This is the region of the brain from where psychomotor seizures usually arise. Surgery consists of the removal of the anterior one-half to two-thirds of the affected lobe (two to three inches). Unfortunately, children with psychomotor seizures which are difficult to control more often than not also have abnormalities in the opposite temporal lobe, or in other areas of the brain, and are thus not good candidates for surgery. If a patient has an epileptogenic focus in both temporal lobes, surgical treatment is not recommended because severe personality changes and loss of memory occur much too frequently when both temporal lobes are removed. No such changes are observed, however, when only one temporal lobe is removed.

Are patients with psychomotor seizures benefited by surgical treatment?

In one study of a large number of patients with psychomotor seizures who were treated surgically and followed for one to twenty-five years, approximately 50 percent had become seizure free, and 25 percent had a marked decrease in the frequency of their seizures. Of the remaining 25 percent, some patients had a less-satisfactory reduction in the frequency of seizures, and in a few the attacks were made worse.

What kind of abnormalities have been found in the temporal lobes of patients undergoing surgery for the treatment of psychomotor seizures?

In most patients who have had a temporal lobectomy, as physicians call this operation, sclerosis (abnormal hardening) of the inner surface of the temporal lobes has been the most common abnormal finding. Other lesions include small congenital benign tumors, scars, and old areas of dead tissue (infarcts) due to lack of blood supply. In about 25 percent of cases, no obvious structural changes have been found.

Have there been any recent advances in the treatment of epilepsy?

Yes. In the past few years medical researchers have developed methods to determine the blood levels of most anticonvulsant drugs in a single blood sample. Also a cerebellar stimulator developed by Dr. Irving S. Cooper and engineer Roger Avery appears to be of value in the treatment of epileptics who do not respond to anticonvulsant drug therapy.

How can the determination of blood levels of anticonvulsants be of help to the child with epilepsy?

Until recently the amount of anticonvulsant given to a child was primarily based on the child's weight and age. This method seemed to work well in most instances. Now we know, however, that in some children even the maximal recommended amount of an anticonvulsant may not produce the blood levels needed to control seizures. Conversely, in some children commonly used dosages may produce high levels and undesirable side effects. It seems that some individuals get rid of the drug too quickly and that others have difficulty in eliminating it. Moreover, the determination of the blood levels of anticonvulsants is an invaluable piece of information when it comes to finding out if an older child is or is not taking his medicine, and in cases of suspected overdose or intoxication.

Unfortunately, at present, facilities for running these tests by a method called "gas liquid chromatography" are available in only a few medical centers. Doubtless when the determination of blood levels of all commonly used anticonvulsants becomes a routine laboratory test, physicians will be able to obtain better control of seizures in a larger number of patients, and at the same time fewer side effects and fewer toxic reactions will occur. Finally, the routine determination of blood levels of a drug a patient is taking may radically change the present methods of prescribing anticonvulsant drugs in three or four daily doses. In the case of Dilantin, for example, researchers have found that blood levels are equally maintained throughout the day irrespective of whether the drug is taken in one, two, or three daily doses. This, of course, may prove eventually to have important practical applications. Most parents are aware that much too often it is difficult to motivate older children to take medications three or four times daily. By the same token, a child of school age may be unwilling or feel ashamed to take his noon dose at school. Once- or twice-daily administration of the drug may be the solution to these very real problems. It should be pointed out that these preliminary reports should not be interpreted as a green light for parents to give anticonvulsants in one single dose to children with seizures. The final decision as to how often during the day anticonvulsant drugs should be administered *has to be made by the prescribing physician* according to the needs of each individual patient.

What about Dr. Irving S. Cooper's procedure of cerebellar stimulation?

Recent reports of Dr. Cooper's work indicate that the surgical implantation of a cerebellar stimulator may be a useful tool in the treatment of patients whose seizures cannot be controlled with drugs. Dr. Cooper's procedure consists in the implantation of two sets of small platinum electrodes over the surface of the cerebellum (the portion of the brain located in the posterior and lower part of the skull). The electrodes are connected by fine wires running under the skin of the neck and chest to a small battery-powered radio transmitter. The procedure is relatively simple and does not involve operating on the brain.

The rationale behind this approach to the treatment of patients with intractable seizures is that electrical stimulation of the cerebellum at certain frequencies appears to have an inhibitory effect on the abnormal electrical discharges causing epileptic seizures. Preliminary results in a small number of patients indicate that cerebellar stimulation may be an important therapeutic tool in the treatment of epilepsy. Of course, only time can tell what the long-term results of this procedure will be.

How often should a child with epilepsy be re-examined by a physician?

It all depends on how easy or how difficult it is to bring his seizures under control. As long as a patient's seizures have not stopped, he should be re-evaluated at frequent intervals, since during this period increments in the dosage of one medication or the addition of new ones will have to be made. Once the patient is free of seizures, he may be re-examined every three or six months. In addition to the physical examination during these follow-up visits, the physician may elect to perform laboratory tests such as a complete blood count, urinalysis, or liver-function tests if the patient is taking a drug which could have adverse effects on the bone marrow, the kidneys, or the liver. Repeat skull x-rays and an electroencephalogram are recommended at yearly intervals in most cases.

Are there any situations in which a child with epilepsy should be hospitalized?

Yes. Even though in most cases a child with seizures can be adequately treated at home, there are several more or less clear-cut indications for hospitalization. As noted in Chapter 1, prolonged grand mal seizures or grand mal seizures occurring in rapid succession (status epilepticus) represent a medical emergency and a potentially lethal situation which require prompt and energetic treatment in a hospital to stop seizure activity. A large number of children are admitted to a hospital following their first grand mal attack. This policy is easy to understand and justify since, although a first convulsion can be the first episode of what eventually will turn out to be a chronic seizure disorder (epilepsy), it can also be the result of acute infections of the brain (encephalitis) or its covering membranes (meningitis), intoxications (lead poisoning, drugs), or the first manifestation of cerebral hemorrhage or a symptom of a disease affecting some other organs of the body. While the child is hospitalized, the physician can perform those tests which have become routine procedures in the diagnostic evaluation of a child with seizures as well as any others that he may consider relevant to any particular situation. We would like to point out that the common policy of hospitalizing a child following a first grand mal seizure is advantageous to the child *medically* and to the parents *economically*. It is a well-known fact that few insurance companies cover physicians' fees or laboratory tests done on an outpatient basis. Most insurance companies, however, will pay anywhere from 70 to 100 percent of the patient's bill as long as the same medical services are provided while the patient is hospitalized. I should emphasize that the decision to hospitalize a child with seizures should, in practically all instances, be made only on medical grounds. The previous statement regarding insurance coverage should not be construed as an advice to take advantage of your insurance policy.

Occasionally it is necessary to hospitalize children for the purpose of substantiating a diagnosis of epileptic seizures. Sometimes the family situation is such that physicians are unable to obtain reliable information from parents regarding the attacks a child may be experiencing. In other cases in which the physician may suspect malingering or hysterical episodes instead of true epileptic seizures, a period of observation in a hospital may be the only way to deal effectively with this dilemma.

As noted previously, the institution of the ketogenic diet in patients with seizures which are resistant to drug therapy is better accomplished in a hospital than at home.

Patients who may be considered to be good candidates for surgical treatment will, of course, need to have a number of studies prior to surgery which can only be performed in a hospital.

In some instances, if a patient continues to have frequent seizures in spite of what appears to be an adequate amount of anticonvulsant, the physician may elect to hospitalize the patient for a period of observation.

In this situation the determination of blood levels of anticonvulsants and the knowledge that the child is indeed taking his medication may provide valuable information. If blood levels are very low in a child whose seizures are not under control in spite of what appears to be an adequate amount of anticonvulsant, there are only three possibilities: the child is not taking his medicine, the drug is not being absorbed in the intestine, or his body is getting rid of it so rapidly after absorption that effective blood concentrations cannot be achieved.

If a patient develops a complication from the administration of an anticonvulsant and a rapid switch to another drug is necessary, the sudden withdrawal of the offending drug is probably safer when done in a hospital, especially if the child has a history of frequent or prolonged grand mal seizures or if he has been taking a drug such as phenobarbital or Dilantin for a fairly prolonged period of time.

How expensive is the treatment of a child with epilepsy?

The medical expenses of parents of children with epilepsy can be considerable. These include not only the regular purchase of one or more medicines but also the cost of blood and urine tests, skull x-rays, and electroencephalograms. The cost of anticonvulsant drugs varies considerably from one child to another according to the type, the amount, and the number of drugs needed to control seizures. The initial medical evaluation done on an outpatient basis can run anywhere from $150 to $250. If the child is hospitalized this amount can easily double. Fortunately, in most cases, electroencephalograms and x-rays, which represent about one-half of this amount, do not have to be repeated more than once a year. In many instances, skull x-rays do not have to be repeated even that frequently. An additional source of expense includes the physician's fees for follow-up visits and the fee for an occasional consultation with a specialist. We can see that in the great majority of cases the cost of treatment of an epileptic child is by no means insignificant. Since many parents cannot afford these expenses, it is recommended that they get in touch with public-health authorities in their community or with representatives of their local chapter of the Epilepsy Foundation to find out whether there are any possible ways to reduce the cost of treatment, follow-up visits to a physician, or laboratory tests. In many states children with epilepsy can obtain financial help from various local or federal agencies. Although children with epilepsy are not crippled individuals, many state legislatures have made them eligible for financial help under the program for crippled children. If parents cannot get financial help from one of the previously mentioned agencies; or if for any reason they are not eligible for it, there is, unfortunately, not much that can be done to reduce the cost of laboratory tests or physicians' fees.

Can anything be done to reduce the cost of anticonvulsant drugs?

Yes. For one thing, the liquid preparations of anticonvulsants are almost always several times more expensive than tablets or capsules. I have mentioned previously that tablets can be given without any difficulty to very young children. Tablets and capsules are not only cheaper than the liquid forms; they are also safer. They say it is cheaper to buy by the dozen. Believe it or not, this rule of thumb also applies to the purchase of drugs. Most anticonvulsants are supplied by drug companies to the pharmacist in bottles of one hundred, five hundred, or one thousand tablets or capsules. The cost of just about any anticonvulsant can be reduced when the number of tablets or capsules prescribed corresponds to the number of units per bottle: 100 or 500, instead of 150 or 250. The reason for this is simple. If by any chance your physician gives you a prescription for 125, 150, or 175 tablets the pharmacist will have to count 25, 50, or 75 tablets from another bottle. This takes time and naturally you will have to pay for it.

There are other ways in which one can cut down on the cost of anticonvulsant drugs. Most anticonvulsants are available in tablets or capsules of different concentrations. Take phenobarbital for example. It is dispensed in tablets containing 1/4, 1/2, 1, and 1 1/2 grains. This is equivalent to 16, 32, 64, and 100 milligrams in the metric system of measure used nowadays by most physicians. It should be pointed out that, whenever a drug, like phenobarbital, is manufactured in tablets of different concentrations, the cost of different tablets is inversely proportional to their concentration. To put this more clearly, 200 quarter-grain tablets are much more expensive than 100 half-grain tablets, although the total amount of drug is exactly the same. If by any chance your child is taking 2 quarter-grain tablets three times a day, ask your physician to give you another prescription so that your child will need to take only 1 half grain tablet three times daily. You may wonder whether children have trouble swallowing a tablet which is twice as strong. None whatsoever. The difference in size is hardly noticeable.

Let's give another example. Valium, a drug widely used

by adults as a sedative, tranquilizer, and muscle relaxant, is at the present time the most effective drug for the treatment of myoclonic and akinetic seizures. Valium comes in tablets of three different concentrations: a white tablet containing two milligrams, a yellow tablet containing five milligrams, and a blue tablet containing ten milligrams. They are all exactly the same size. Valium is an expensive drug. For this reason, and whenever possible, we have made it a custom to prescribe this drug in the more-concentrated tablet forms. For example, if a child needs to take six milligrams of Valium three times a day, instead of writing a prescription for two-milligram tablets we prescribe two different tablet forms, one for five-milligram tablets and another one for two-milligram tablets, and tell the parents to give the child one five-milligram tablet and one-half of the two-milligram tablet (equals six milligrams). Again, by following this policy both the child as well as the parents will benefit. The parents will save some money and the child will need to take only one and one-half tablets instead of three tablets three times a day. The same type of prescribing gymnastics can be done with most, although not all, anticonvulsant drugs presently available. Another helpful suggestion to reduce the cost of drugs is to find out the cost of your prescription before having it filled. You will be surprised to know to what extent the price of medicines varies from one pharmacy to another. In case you are not aware of it, the price of drugs is not subject to any kind of state or federal control or regulation. As long as you are willing to pay, the pharmacist is entitled to charge you as much as he wishes. In our community at least, the cost of some anticonvulsants vary as much as 50 to 75 percent in different pharmacies. We should also mention that the same holds true for just about any other medication available only on prescription.

6. What Is the Prognosis
for a Child with Epilepsy?

Does epilepsy get worse with age?

No. In the overwhelming majority of cases seizures do not get worse with advancing age. On the contrary, it is well known that some types of seizures which occur only in infancy and early childhood tend to decrease in frequency or to cease completely as the child gets older. Febrile seizures are a good example of a type of seizure that decreases in frequency or severity and eventually disappears altogether with increasing age. Febrile seizures are a very common problem during the first five years of life, seldom occur after the age of six, and never after the age of seven years. Somehow aging, and the cerebral maturation which goes along with it, appear to take care of them. Although the overwhelming majority of children with febrile seizures are not epileptics, their decreased brain resistance to the development of seizures with febrile illnesses and the subsequent increase of this resistance with cerebral maturation are a good example of the point I'm trying to make. Petit mal, a type of epilepsy which almost always begins between the ages of four and ten years, also has the tendency to decrease in severity after the age of puberty and seldom persists beyond the age of twenty years.

In a rare instance, however, seizures are not only impossible to control with any form of treatment presently available, but actually do get worse as the child gets older. They can become more frequent, more severe, or both. It should be pointed out, however, that this is the exception rather than the rule.

Dr. William Lennox, a pioneer in the study of epilepsy in the United States, has written the following in regard to seizures and age:* "Another natural, although unpopular, chemical inhibitor of seizures is the process of aging. Explanation for this healing influence is not yet forthcoming, but the observation that brain waves become faster and more stabilized and that the abnormal electrical pulsations of epilepsy as well as the surface seizures tend to become fewer [with age] is well recognized."

What are the odds that a child who receives adequate anticonvulsant treatment will "outgrow" his seizures and that eventually he will be able to get along without having to take medicines?

It has been estimated that in about 75 percent of epileptic children who have been free of seizures for more than three years, and in whom treatment is discontinued, seizures will not recur. This leaves us with 25 percent of epileptic children in whom recurrence of seizures can be expected following withdrawal of medications. In this regard, children fare much better than adults. This 25 percentage is only half as great as the rate of seizure recurrence in adults after withdrawal of medicine following a seizure-free interval of three years.

What can be done if seizures should recur?

If seizures recur, and the chances are that they will recur in one out of four children, treatment with the anticonvulsant

* William G. Lennox, M.A., "Therapeutics of Epilepsy," *Therapeutic Notes* 61, no. 5 (May 1954): 134.

previously used should be reinstituted immediately after the first seizure.

Is there a way to predict which child is most likely to remain free of seizures after medication is discontinued?

Although there are no reliable ways of predicting whether a patient will remain seizure-free after medication is withdrawn, there are certain factors, such as the age at which seizures began and the ease with which they can be brought under control, that may allow physicians to make a fairly accurate estimate concerning the chances of seizure recurrence. For example, when seizures begin early in life (before the age of two years), the chance of recurrence is less than when they begin after the age of two years. The older the child at the time of his first seizure, the closer he approaches the chance of recurrence seen in adult epileptics. By the same token, when seizures are easy to control at the beginning of treatment, the better the outlook regarding possible recurrence at a later age. Neither sex, race, frequency, severity of attacks, nor a family history of epilepsy appears to be an important factor in predicting whether seizures will recur after withdrawal of anticonvulsant medications. The age at the time of drug withdrawal does not seem to correlate well with seizure recurrence.

For many years the medical literature has suggested that there is a high risk of recurrence when anticonvulsant drugs are withdrawn at the time of puberty, especially in females. Recent reports indicate this may be an unjustified fear. Nevertheless, because the influence of hormonal changes of puberty on the brain are still largely unknown, most physicians recommend withdrawal of drugs in pubertal females after a seizure-free interval of at least three years, and only after menstrual periods have become regular.

Are the chances of "outgrowing" seizures with appropriate treatment more or less the same for different types?

No. Following drug withdrawal, the lowest incidence of seizure recurrence is seen in patients with grand mal and petit mal. Children with focal, myoclonic, or akinetic seizures and those who have more than one type of attack appear to have the poorest outlook. The prognosis for patients with psychomotor attacks lies somewhere in between those with grand mal and those with focal motor seizures. The chances of seizure recurrence after withdrawal of medication is about twice as high in children with severe physical or mental handicaps as in those who have no major physical or mental problems.

What is the life expectancy of an epileptic child?

In the overwhelming majority of cases, it is not different from that of a "normal" person. For a number of years textbooks of medicine and articles published in medical journals contended that the life expectancy of epileptics is considerably less than that of the general population. Most of the studies quoted to support this statement were conducted in institutionalized patients who, in addition to having seizures, suffered from severe physical and mental handicaps due to a variety of causes. Today most physicians agree that, with the exception of children with myoclonic seizures beginning early in infancy (a type of epilepsy which is in almost 100 percent of cases associated with severe and often progressive physical and mental deterioration), life expectancy in the rest of epileptics does not differ in any significant way from that of the so-called "normal" population.

In this regard we should point out that statistics can sometimes be exceedingly misleading. Take, for example, the figures concerning the life expectancy of the average American. Statisticians tell us that life expectancy in this country has increased from about fifty years in 1900 to approximately seventy years in 1972. If one considers the methods by which statisticians have arrived at these figures, it becomes quite clear that this is not entirely as it appears. Life expectancy in this country has not truly increased twenty-five years during the course of this century. What statisticians fail to tell us is that in 1900 life expectancy was fifty years because for each individual who reached old age there was another who died during the first month or first year of life. We often read in newspapers or magazines that life expectancy in certain underdeveloped countries is thirty-two or thirty-five years. If you happen to visit one of these countries, you will be surprised to see that the largest percentage of the population consists of old and not young people.

Unfortunately the same general principles have been applied by statisticians when attempting to determine the longevity of epileptics: the child with severe physical and mental handicaps, and who also happens to have seizures, has been lumped together with the average epileptic, whose life span is similar to that of the nonepileptic. It is inevitable that when two entirely different population samples are put together, a strong bias is introduced and the result can be nothing but a meaningless figure.

Parents of epileptic children should know that seizures *per se* are an extremely rare cause of premature death; that with adequate treatment, and probably even without the benefit of it, the mortality risk is not greater than in the average person; and that there is no reason why a child with epilepsy should not live as long as he would were he not an epileptic.

How often is it necessary to institutionalize an epileptic child?

Epilepsy *per se* is rarely, if ever, a valid reason for placing a child in an institution. The indications for institutionalization of a child with epilepsy fall into three categories: (1) when he suffers from profound mental retardation as a result of severe congenital developmental defects of the brain or as a consequence of serious brain injuries sustained at the time of birth or in early infancy, (2) in those extremely rare cases in which the child has exceedingly severe and frequent (daily) seizures which are resistant to all types of treatment, and (3) in the rare case of an adolescent, usually suffering from psychomotor seizures, who has a behavior or a psychiatric problem of such magnitude that it makes it impossible for him to live according to the rules and laws of society.

7. Is There Any Relationship Between Epilepsy and Mental Retardation?

Is there any relationship between epilepsy and mental retardation?

It all depends on how one looks at the problem. If one wishes to be precise and accurate, the answer must be an emphatic *NO*. Epilepsy is by no means incompatible with average or above average intelligence.

Since by definition epilepsy is not a specific disease but the outward manifestation of intermittent, short-lasting disturbances in the electrical activity of the brain due to a wide variety of causes, if any relationship exists between epilepsy and mental retardation it would have to be not with the seizures *per se* but with whatever is the cause of them. If seizures are due to severe brain defects or are due to severe birth trauma or birth asphyxia, or are the result of encephalitis or meningitis during early infancy or childhood, the chances of associated mental retardation will have to be, of necessity, greater than in those children in whom the cause of epilepsy is the abnormal functioning of only a small group of brain cells.

If one keeps in mind the concept that epilepsy is merely a symptom of periodic abnormal cerebral function, and that seizures *per se* will only in extremely rare instances cause mental deterioration in a child who is of average intelligence, or produce further mental regression in one who is mentally retarded, we can dogmatically state that epilepsy does not cause mental retardation, but instead that a certain number of mentally retarded children also happen to suffer from epilepsy. A number of well-known historical figures who are said to have suffered from epilepsy were nonetheless capable of great achievements at a time when there was no effective treatment. Among these prominent personalities there were statesmen (Julius Caesar, Peter the Great, Napoleon Bonaparte), religious leaders (Buddha, Mohammed, St. Paul), literary men (Lord Byron, Dostoyevsky, Flaubert, Guy de Maupassant), famous composers (Handel, Berlioz), philosophers and mathematicians (Socrates, Pascal), and many others.

Whether or not all these famous people were indeed epileptic will probably always remain a matter of speculation. The biographical information on which a retrospective diagnosis of epilepsy has been made is in some cases scanty, and in others difficult to accept in line with present medical knowledge.

Julius Caesar apparently had at least two well-documented grand mal episodes during the African campaigns. On several occasions, Napoleon Bonaparte is said to have experienced attacks during which his face became distorted, he lost consciousness and fell to the ground.

St. Paul's fall from his horse on his way to Damascus and his temporary blindness for the following three days could very well have been a cerebral concussion or, as suggested by Dr. William Lennox, a severe attack of migraine (sick headache).

Peter the Great, Czar of Russia, on the other hand, did have fairly frequent epileptic seizures. So did his half-brother, Ivan. Lord Byron had several episodes of what present-day physicians would not hesitate to call a psychomotor seizure. There is little doubt that Dostoyevsky, the great Russian novelist, also had psychomotor epilepsy and that he experienced fairly frequent attacks.

How do children with epilepsy compare in intelligence with nonepileptic children?

Extremely well. In general, the intelligence of persons with epilepsy more or less parallels that of the general population. Some are retarded or dull, the great majority have average intellectual abilities, and some are of superior intelligence.

When discussing the relationship between epilepsy and intelligence a distinction should be made between children who have primary epilepsy and those affected with secondary epilepsy. As a group the intelligence of children with primary or idiopathic (unknown cause) epilepsy does not differ significantly from that of nonepileptic children. On the other hand, children with secondary or acquired epilepsy whose seizures are a manifestation of a structural lesion of the brain have, as a group, less than average intelligence when compared with the normal population. Since the incidence of mental retardation in children with secondary or acquired epilepsy is relatively high, in any large randomly selected group of children with epilepsy one is bound to find an incidence of mental retardation approximately three to four times higher than in the general population. These figures, however, are considerably smaller than those that by word of mouth and in popular magazines have been passed from one generation to the next. In the past it was believed that all epileptics were mentally retarded. Misconceptions in this respect arose from studies conducted in small groups of institutionalized patients who suffered from severe mental retardation and who also happened to have seizures. It is obvious that in such a selected and biased population sample the incidence of mental deficiency among epileptics will be very high, and the incidence of epilepsy among the mentally deficient will also be very high. It just couldn't be any other way.

We should re-emphasize here the fundamental concept that epilepsy is not a specific disease, but is only a symptom or manifestation of transient abnormalities in cerebral function. A child cannot be mentally retarded because he has epilepsy. If he is mentally retarded, whatever is causing his mental retardation is more than likely, in one way or another, also to be the cause of his seizures.

Is there any relationship between seizure type and intelligence?

Yes. There is little doubt that to a certain extent a relationship does exist between type of seizure and intelligence. We mentioned above that patients who have so-called primary epilepsy (some forms of grand mal and all petit mal) compare favorably with the population at large in terms of intelligence. The same is also true of most patients who suffer from psychomotor seizures. On the other hand, patients with minor motor seizures (myoclonic and akinetic) are as a group less intelligent than patients with other types of seizures. Here the words "as a group" should be emphasized. In any large group of patients with this type of seizure one will find some who are of average or above average intelligence. However, the number of those with less than average intelligence will be higher when compared to children with other types of seizures or to children from the general population.

Finally, an almost direct relationship exists between seizures and mental development in children in whom minor motor seizures, especially myoclonic, begin during the first two years of life. The chance of normal mental development in these children is very small. The overwhelming majority of them (more than 95 percent) have severe mental retardation and eventually will need to be institutionalized. Fortunately, minor motor seizures starting in early infancy account for only a small percentage of all cases of epilepsy in childhood. As previously noted, the cause of the slow mental development in these children is *not the seizures* but whatever is causing them. Even though in the great majority of these children seizures can be brought under complete control with appropriate treatment, the basic process which caused both the mental retardation and the seizures remains unchanged.

Since my child had a grand mal convulsion at six months of age I'm terribly conscious of his development. Deep down I cannot help but feel that either the convulsion or the medicine he has to take every day will slow him down. How can I know that this is not happening to him?

There is little evidence to support the belief that short-lasting grand mal seizures *per se* will cause deterioration of a child's intellectual abilities. It is possible that brief periods of cerebral hypoxia (lack of oxygen) at the beginning of a grand mal seizure may damage a small number of brain cells. If something of this nature does indeed occur, it must be of such small magnitude that in the overwhelming majority of cases it cannot be demonstrated by our present method of testing a child's intelligence. To put it in other words, if a child has an IQ of one hundred at the age of three years and for the next four years has x number of seizures, the chances that his IQ will remain unchanged are excellent. In rare occasions, a child may show signs of mental regression after suffering from prolonged grand mal seizures or status epilepticus. We mentioned earlier that status epilepticus is a medical emergency which requires prompt and energetic treatment. It is obvious then that a child who recovers from a potentially fatal condition may well be left with irreversible brain damage. In the majority of instances, however, no such damage occurs. Many years of experience have also shown that the daily administration of anticonvulsant medications has no handicapping effect on the child's psychomotor development.

As a general frame of reference we have listed in Appendix 2 the most important milestones of psychomotor (mental-physical) development during the first six years of life. When using this table as a guide for a child's development, it should be kept in mind that mental retardation is sometimes difficult to recognize during the first six months of life. Unless severe birth defects are present, mental retardation can easily go unsuspected until an infant fails to reach certain well-known milestones of motor development such as sitting without support, pulling up to stand, or walking. In an older infant (twelve to eighteen months) with normal motor development, mental retardation can also go undetected until he fails to acquire speech at the expected age. Milestones of motor and mental development are usually equally impaired in mentally retarded children. Motor milestones have a much wider range of normal variation than mental milestones, which tend to appear at a more or less constant age. It is not too uncommon, for example, to see a child of normal intelligence who does not sit until eight or nine months of age or one who does not walk unaided until the age of eighteen months. It is rare, on the other hand, to see a normal infant who does not smile before the age of two months, one who in the absence of physical handicap does not adopt a position of welcome to his mother's presence by the age of four to five months, or an infant older than six months who does not cry when left alone with strangers. By the same token, parents as well as physicians have to be alerted to the possibility of mental retardation or hearing deficit if a child does not say his first meaningful word by eighteen months of age.

What about infants who are just late talkers? Isn't it true that sometimes slow speech development runs in families?

Yes. Sometimes it does. But we should also remember that exceptions only serve to confirm the rule. It is true that occasionally one sees a normal child who does not walk until the age of two years, or one who does not say his first meaningful single word until the age of seventeen or eighteen months and whose parents, or at least one of whose parents, was also slow in walking or talking. We should point out, however, that at least in our experience this is not a very common occurrence. We have made it a custom, therefore, whenever we see a child who has not said his first single word by eighteen months of age to make every possible effort to determine whether there is any medical reason to account for his delayed speech development.

Is a child who doesn't talk at the expected age always retarded?

Not necessarily. Actually, the most common cause of slow speech development is not mental retardation. It is deafness. Furthermore, hearing loss does not need to amount to total deafness to be a cause of retarded speech development. A child with a hearing loss for high frequency sounds (consonants, for example) will be unable to reproduce speech sounds even if he's able to respond to sounds of low frequencies, such as those produced by many musical toys, the ringing of a telephone, or the dropping of a heavy object on the floor. These considerations only emphasize the need for justified concern on the part of both parents and physicians when confronted with a child who appears to be slow in acquiring speech when compared with other children of the same age.

What if a child was a premature baby?

An entirely different situation exists if the child was born prematurely. Premature babies do not reach the milestones of psychomotor development at the ages indicated in Appendix 2. The great majority of normal premature babies are able to catch up rapidly with normal full-term babies in terms of motor and mental development. Nevertheless, at least during the first year and a half of life, all premature babies should be given credit for their prematurity. In other words, if an infant was three months premature he should not be expected to reach the milestones of psychomotor development until he is three months older than the figures for full-term babies listed in Appendix 2. The same rule applies if the baby was one or two months premature. By the end of the second year of life, the normal premature baby, irrespective of his degree of prematurity, has almost always caught up with the average full-term baby and therefore his abilities (mental and physical) should now be compared with those of the average child.

If our child has not reached the milestones of development at the expected age how do we know whether he is retarded or whether he is just slow?

This is invariably the first question parents ask their physician after telling him that their child is already nine months of age and doesn't sit without help, or that he is eighteen months of age and still is unable to utter a single word.

We mentioned above that milestones of motor development vary considerably from one child to another, but that the same is not true of mental milestones which are reached at more or less predictable ages. The fact that a child has reached the motor milestones of development at the anticipated age is by no means a guarantee that his mental development will also be normal. On the other hand, it is not at all uncommon to see infants and young children who, because of some type of physical handicap, may be considerably behind in motor development and still are average or above average in mental development. This marked discrepancy between motor and mental development is frequently observed, for example, in children suffering from cerebral palsy, or in those who have some other type of physical handicap.

If a child is significantly behind in mental development, even if his motor development is normal, he should not be labeled as just a "slow child," if by this it is meant that sooner or later he will be able to catch up with the average child. A major source of confusion that parents have regarding the words "retarded" and "slow" appears to derive from the erroneous idea of thinking about mental development in months or years rather than in terms of developmental quotient (months or years of retardation in relation to the age of the child). Time and again we see parents who are genuinely convinced that their child is only six or twelve months behind in his psychomotor development when in fact he may have a developmental quotient of fifty or less. For example, a twelve-month-old infant functioning at a six-month level of psychomotor development is not really six months "behind" as compared to a normal twelve-month-old infant, but 50 percent of his life behind, so that when he reaches the age of twelve years chances are that his mental age will be six years and not eleven and a half years. It is then not difficult to realize why in the minds of so many parents to be six months "behind" seems to be a rather minor delay which the infant or young child may easily make up for within the next year or so. Unfortunately, in the great majority of cases this "catching up" just does not occur.

Could you repeat the same thing in simpler words? I didn't quite understand the previous example. If a seven-year-old child is two years behind in his development, he should be able to function as well as a five-year-old. Right?

Right.

So that, instead of finishing high school at age seventeen he'll finish at age nineteen. Right?

Wrong.

Why is that?

Simply because people reach their adult intelligence levels at approximately age fourteen, give or take six or twelve months. After age fourteen people may acquire new knowledge, sometimes a tremendous amount of it, but that doesn't make them more intelligent. Therefore, if a child is two years behind in his mental development at age seven, all that means is that his IQ is about eighty, which is not high enough to succeed in an average elementary school. And by the time he's fourteen his IQ will still be eighty, not enough to compete in senior high. Now, if a child is two years behind at age four, his IQ is about fifty, which means he'll never be able to lead an independent life and should be seriously considered for institutionalization.

8. Is Epilepsy Inherited?

Is epilepsy hereditary?

In more than one way, yes. But so many factors appear to be involved for the condition to be passed on from one generation to another that, for all practical purposes, nobody needs to worry too much about it. As we will later see, the chance that a parent with epilepsy may pass on the condition to his descendants, or that parents with an affected child may have a second affected child, is not much higher than those of "normal" parents.

Since antiquity epilepsy has been considered to be an inherited disorder. Hippocrates, the great physician of ancient Greece, mentioned in his monograph "On the Sacred Disease" (400 B.C.) that epilepsy "was a disease of the brain" and that "its origins are hereditary." Whether or not genetic factors play a significant role in epilepsy has been the subject of a great deal of controversy among contemporary specialists in epilepsy and genetics. Over the past twenty years opinions in this regard have varied considerably. Some investigators have postulated that heredity plays a relatively important role in certain forms of epilepsy such as petit mal and primary or idiopathic (of unknown cause) grand mal. A second group of investigators, on the other hand, believe that heredity probably plays no role whatever in epilepsy. Finally, a third

149

and more eclectic group have adopted a middle-of-the-road position and maintain that at the present time the hereditary transmission of epilepsy cannot be demonstrated nor can it be ruled out entirely. Dr. Samuel Livingston, one of the best-known epileptologists in the U.S.A., after analyzing the many studies conducted by a fairly large number of investigators on the genetics of epilepsy, including his own study, concludes that a clear-cut genetic mode of transmission of epilepsy has so far not been definitely established. He states that at the present time a number of authorities in the fields of epilepsy and genetics believe that the inheritance of epilepsy has not been proved and that the data compiled to date would indicate that the genetic factor in epilepsy is slight. We should add, however, that no matter how slight this factor may be, it is responsible for a higher risk of epilepsy in families in which one member is already affected, especially when the involved individual has primary or idiopathic epilepsy.

In spite of such divergent opinions it is generally agreed that a predisposition to develop epilepsy appears to be inherited. A similar inherited predisposition has been demonstrated in certain other diseases such as diabetes and high blood pressure. It is well known that not all persons who are born with a predisposition to develop a particular disease will indeed develop the disease. In some patients with diabetes, for example, environmental factors such as a high-carbohydrate diet and excessive weight are needed for the inherited predisposition to produce the clinical symptoms of the disease.

What does it mean to say that a person may inherit a tendency or predisposition to develop seizures?

In general, what a person may inherit is not a particular type of epilepsy but a predisposition that means he will have a lesser degree of resistance than the average individual to developing seizures under similar unfavorable circumstances (brain injury, fever, etc.). We have already pointed out that this lesser degree of resistance or low seizure threshold explains why, of two persons with exactly the same type of brain injury, one will and the other will not develop seizures. I said in Chapter 1 that the ability to convulse is an intrinsic quality of the human brain and that in this respect, and given the right circumstances, no one is exempt. It is also true, however, that there is a great deal of variation from one person to another in terms of their readiness to convulse under similar adverse conditions, or following a similar or identical brain injury.

If my husband or I have epilepsy what are the chances that one or more of our children will also be affected? And if one of our children has epilepsy, what is the risk that we may also have other affected children?

The chances are different according to the type of epilepsy. If the cause of seizures in a parent or a child is an injury to the brain due to organic causes such as birth trauma or meningitis (secondary epilepsy), the chances that the parents may have one or more affected children are only slightly higher than in the general population. On first thought this just doesn't make any sense. It seems totally illogical to assume that inheritance should play a role in the development of seizures when these are due to an injury or an infection occurring during the early development of an individual. By the same token it is difficult to believe that such an affected individual could be able to pass an acquired condition to his descendants. The situation, however, is not that simple. It appears that even in cases of secondary or acquired epilepsy, a hereditary predisposition—manifested as a lower brain resistance to the development of seizures—also plays a role. In other words, the injury or illness that triggers seizures in individuals with a genetic predisposition to epilepsy is less likely to cause seizures in an individual without this genetic factor. This would explain why only a certain number of children who recover from diseases such as meningitis, encephalitis, brain abscesses or other diseases affecting the brain will subsequently develop seizures, and would also explain why only about 20 percent of soldiers with similar head injuries sustained during World War II eventually became epileptics. Admittedly the chances of having another affected child when a previous sibling is affected with secondary or acquired epilepsy are small. Unless similar circumstances (birth trauma, infections of the brain, etc.) are present, the risk that a couple will have a second child also affected is probably not significantly higher than that of other couples who have not had an affected child.

On the other hand, when it comes to primary or idiopathic epilepsy, the type which is characterized by intermittent episodes of abnormal cerebral function in spite of entirely normal cerebral architecture, the opinion of most investigators is that inheritance plays a relatively important role.

According to the extensive studies conducted by Dr. Julius Metrakos and Dr. Katherine Metrakos, the risk of epilepsy of primary or idiopathic (unknown) origin for a child who has an affected parent or sibling is as indicated in Appendix 3.

If a child has a parent or a sibling with primary epilepsy, the risk that he will also develop seizures is 8 percent. If in one family there is a parent and a sibling affected with epilepsy, the risk that a second child may also be affected increases to 13 percent. If one sibling is affected but both parents are normal the risk is slightly smaller (7 percent) than the overall basic risk of 8 percent.

The risk that a child who has either an affected parent or an affected sibling will also develop epilepsy varies with the age of onset of seizures in the involved relative. If the onset of seizures in the parent or sibling was before the age of two and one-half years the chances that a child or another sibling will also be involved is higher (10 percent) than if the onset in the affected relative was after the age of two and one-half years (6 percent).

As illustrated in Appendix 3, the overall basic risk decreases as a child gets older, from 6 percent at age one, to 2 percent by age six, and to less than 1 percent by age ten. This simply means that if a parent or sibling has primary epilepsy the risk that a subsequent child will also develop seizures decreases as he gets older, to the point that, by the time he reaches the age of twelve years, there is for all practical purposes no risk.

If one identical twin is affected with primary epilepsy, the risk that the other twin will also develop seizures is about 80 to 90 percent. The risk for nonidentical (fraternal) twins is not different from that of ordinary siblings.

Is there any way to predict whether a child who has a parent or a sibling with primary epilepsy will or will not be affected?

Yes. In this particular situation, if electroencephalograms performed at periodic intervals (usually yearly) between the ages of five and fifteen years are normal, there is less than a 1 percent risk that the child will develop epilepsy. If the electroencephalogram shows the same type of abnormalities as those present in the affected parent or sibling, the risk increases to the overall basic risk of 8 percent.

Isn't an overall risk of 8 percent a rather high figure?

It all depends on the way one looks at it. If a parent has primary epilepsy or normal parents already have an affected child, the chances of *not having* a first or second child with seizures is 92 percent. Doubtless this is a much more optimistic and by no means a less realistic way of looking at the problem.

As previously mentioned, if in a given family a parent or a sibling suffers from secondary (acquired) epilepsy the risk of having a first or a second affected sibling is much less than 8

percent, probably only slightly higher than the risk of epilepsy in children of normal parents, which is about 2 percent.

**If one parent suffers from an inherited disease, one of whose
symptoms is epileptic seizures, or if both parents are carriers
of the gene of a similar disease, what are the chances that one
or more of their children will be affected?**

In less than 0.5 percent of children with epilepsy, seizures
are only one of several symptoms of a disease which the child
has inherited either from one or from both parents. If, in
addition to carrying genes for the disease, one of the parents
also manifests symptoms of the disease, the chance that the
offspring—sons or daughters—will inherit the disease is 50
percent with each pregnancy. From a genetic standpoint,
diseases which are transmitted in this way, such as some forms
of muscular dystrophy, are called autosomal dominant. On
the other hand, if the parents are "apparently" normal, but
both are carriers of the abnormal gene (hereditary unit) for
a particular disease, the chance of having an affected child is
25 percent with each pregnancy. This mode of inheritance
is called autosomal recessive. The overwhelming majority of
inherited diseases affecting the nervous system (phenylketonuria, Tay-Sachs disease, and a number of other conditions associated either with seizures or mental retardation)
of man are transmitted in this manner. As noted above, however, in only a very small percentage (less than 0.5 percent)
of all children with epilepsy is the condition due to inherited
diseases affecting the nervous system.

**Where should parents go for genetic counseling if one of
them or one of their children has or has had epilepsy?**

From the preceding comments it is clear that whoever
makes a diagnosis of epilepsy (pediatrician, neurologist, etc.)
and, on the basis of the clinical history of the child, the find-

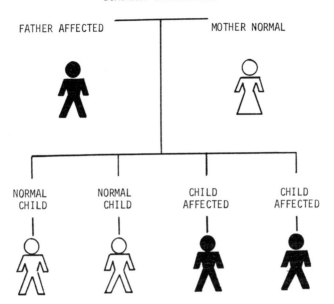

Fig. 6. Autosomal Dominant Inheritance

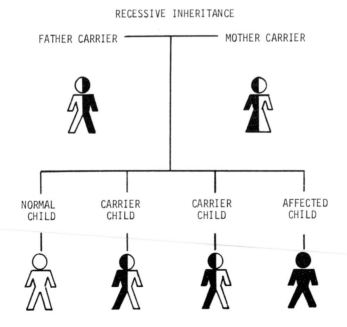

Fig. 7. Autosomal Recessive Dominance

ings of the physical examination, and the results of laboratory
tests, determines what type of epilepsy a child has, is the right
person from whom to obtain genetic advice. We have to admit that genetic counseling can be, at best, a vague exercise
in statistics as well as a frustrating experience for both parents
and physicians. As pointed out by the Metrakos', "What do
statistics and probabilities mean to a parent who is concerned
not with the average of 100 children but with a specific child
—a son or daughter?"

**What would you do if you yourself had epilepsy or if you had
a child affected with epilepsy?**

I don't think I would worry too much about it. Not that
I don't believe in statistics. Far from that. It is unrealistic to
dismiss statistics and probabilities as merely abstract concepts.
They are a fact of life and they are here to stay, reminding us
every single day of our lives of their very concrete existence.
We know, for example, that 3 to 5 percent of babies born
every day will be mentally retarded, that 15 percent of them
will have serious learning difficulties in spite of having
average intelligence, and that perfectly normal parents have
a 2 percent chance of having a child with epilepsy. We also
know that approximately five hundred persons die each year
during the Labor Day weekend as a result of automobile
accidents. We have no choice but to face the fact that every
day of our lives, and whether we like it or not, all of us have
to take a number of risks. Since there isn't much that we can
do about it, the sooner we convince ourselves that they are
worth taking, the better. What I'm really trying to say is that
the chances of not having a child affected with epilepsy, when
one parent or one child is affected, are so heavily in favor of
the parents that I believe it is a risk worth taking.

9. Living with an Epileptic Child

What can parents do at the time of an attack?

In contrast to popular belief, unless very special circumstances are present there isn't much that anybody can do to stop a seizure. Old rituals used in the "revival" of a person who has fainted—applying cold water to the face or trying to pour water or any other kind of liquid down the mouth will do nothing to stop a seizure or shorten its duration. The latter procedure should be avoided; it will be of no benefit to the child and can be dangerous. A large portion of the liquid may go down the windpipe and into his lungs instead of his stomach. It is only when the child happens to be in a hospital, has an intravenous drip going, and a physician is at the bedside with a syringeful of anticonvulsant in his hand, that the duration of an attack may be shortened.

The great majority of grand mal seizures have long subsided before the child is taken to a physicians's office or to the emergency room of a hospital. Other types of seizures last a considerably shorter time than the classic grand mal attack. Still, there are a few things that any person can do to help a child during the course of a grand mal attack. I should mention here that the seizure *per se*, or more precisely the changes which are taking place in the brain at the time of a seizure, are usually of no great significance. Therefore, any measures one may take to help the child are primarily designed to prevent problems arising from the external manifestations of an attack, such as the loss of consciousness, the jerking of the extremities, and the tightening of the muscles of the jaw. The following measures, therefore, are intended to prevent external injuries and for obvious reason apply only to grand mal seizures.

Get the child in a position where he will not hurt himself by knocking his jerking extremities against something. Remember that you cannot stop the muscle jerking, so don't try to interfere with his movements. Loosen tight clothing, especially around the neck. If the child is at home during an attack, he can be laid down on a soft surface. If he is at school, the same objective can be accomplished by putting him on the floor with a pillow or a coat under his head to prevent injury on a hard floor. To avoid tongue or cheek biting, a folded handkerchief or a piece of cloth can be slipped between the upper and lower jaw, but only if the child's mouth is not yet tightly closed. Do not use hard objects such as a spoon or not-too-hard but sensitive objects such as your index finger. A spoon can produce unnecessary damage to the child's teeth or mouth; the finger can leave *you* in a painful situation. After a child's first seizure, the parents or the school nurse can make an excellent padded gag with a wooden tongue depressor, a piece of gauze and adhesive tape, and have it on hand for future seizures. Once the spell is over, let him rest or sleep if he wants to.

Children with petit mal or minor motor seizures (myoclonic and akinetic) usually do not require any special treatment. These seizures are associated with only momentary loss of awareness or very brief loss of consciousness. They seldom last more than a few seconds, and if the child falls to the ground during a minor motor seizure he gets up and returns to his normal self almost immediately. In most cases the best way to handle a child having a psychomotor seizure is to let him continue his "unusual activity" without verbal or forceful restraint. Remember again that nothing you might tell him or do to him, such as slapping his face, shaking his body, or applying cold water to his face, will stop the duration or change the nature of the seizure.

Can a child swallow his tongue during a grand mal seizure?

No, he cannot. During a grand mal seizure the throat muscles are drawn so tight that it is impossible for him to swallow anything, even his tongue.

What should parents do after a child has had a grand mal seizure?

The answer to this question depends primarily on whether the seizure is the first episode or is one of several a child has had over a certain period of time. If a child is known to have epilepsy, the occurrence of another seizure, as a rule, does not represent an emergency situation. The physician taking care of the child usually has advised the parents about what to do should another seizure occur. He may have told them to get in touch with him over the phone or to bring the child to his office, or he may have advised them to increase the amount of drug the child is taking. In this regard we must again emphasize that parents should not increase the amount of an anticonvulsant drug if the physician has not given them such advice. They should remember that the child may already be taking the maximal amount of drug that he can tolerate for his age and weight and, consequently, that an increase in dosage may produce toxic effects.

An entirely different situation exists when a child has his first grand mal seizure and there is no way of knowing just by its nature or duration whether it represents the first epi-sode of what eventually will turn out to be a chronic seizure disorder (epilepsy) or whether it is due to acute illnesses affecting the brain or other organs. A first seizure has to be differentiated from a host of other conditions, such as encephalitis, meningitis, intoxications, and acute kidney problems, disorders whose initial symptom may be a grand mal seizure. Because these are all very real possibilities, it is mandatory that a child be examined by a physician shortly after his first grand mal seizure in order to rule out a fairly large number of diagnostic possibilities such as those mentioned above.

If a first grand mal seizure is a symptom of an acute disease affecting either the brain or other organs, it is obvious that we are dealing with a problem which, at least at this time, is not epilepsy. We say "at least at this time" because there are a fairly large number of acute diseases affecting the brain which can produce changes that eventually lead to epilepsy.

Can other types of seizures also represent emergency situations?

Rarely, if ever. It is always possible that a first psychomotor seizure may be the initial manifestation of a brain tumor arising from one temporal lobe of the brain. If the child appears to be back to normal after the seizure is over the situation is certainly not an emergency. The same is true of petit mal, myoclonic, akinetic, or convulsive equivalent attacks. As a matter of fact, we cannot remember more than one or two children with any of these forms of epilepsy who were taken to a physician shortly after their first attack. We have mentioned previously that, due to the clinical characteristics of these attacks, they may easily go unrecognized for quite some time before their true epileptic nature is suspected. Not infrequently weeks, and occasionally months, may elapse before the parents of many of these children seek medical attention.

Should parents take the child to a hospital after each seizure recurrence?

If you happen to know that your physician is readily available in the emergency room of a nearby hospital, by all means. Otherwise, it is always better to try to get in touch with him over the phone and explain the situation to him or follow the instructions he has already given you should such a situation arise. Generally, if a child has a seizure similar to the ones he has had in the past, there is no reason for undue concern or alarm. A word of caution, however, is in order here. Common sense indicates that children with epilepsy are not immune to other illnesses whose initial symptom may be a seizure. It is advisable then that parents immediately get in touch with their physician if a child has a seizure recurrence in association with manifestations which have not been present during previous attacks such as high fever, severe and prolonged headache, deterioration of the level of consciousness of a severity and duration different from those experienced previously, or any other symptoms which do not seem to fit the regular pattern of his seizures.

Should parents keep an exact written record of a child's seizures?

My personal opinion is that in most instances this is not necessary. This doesn't mean that parents shouldn't keep an accurate record, mental or written, of what happens to their child *during* an attack. But it is the nature of the attacks and their approximate duration which is of diagnostic importance to the physician. I'm aware that a number of seizure clinics as well as many physicians give parents especially designed forms so that they can keep as accurate a record as possible of all seizures a child may have, including the exact time of the day at which they occur, and their exact duration. Unless both parents suffer from a pathologically poor memory, we do not recommend the keeping of a precise daily or weekly written record of all the seizures a child may have over a certain period of time. I believe that this practice is an unnecessary exercise in compulsion and, in most cases, an unjustified emotional burden on the parents. If parents are unduly preoccupied with the recording of irrelevant written infomation, they may be able to provide the physician with accurate statistical minutiae and be totally unable to tell him what actually happens to their child during a seizure. Since the goal in the medical treatment of an epileptic child is to bring his seizures under complete control, as long as he is having frequent attacks he will have to be re-examined at fairly frequent intervals. For the treating physician, it doesn't really make much difference if the frequency of petit mal seizures decreases from thirty to twenty a day or the frequency of psychomotor seizures from six to four a week following the beginning of therapy. Adjustments in the dosage of one drug or the administration of new ones will have to be made irrespective of a slight or moderate decrease in the number of attacks. On the other hand, if a child's seizures decrease in frequency from thirty to one a day or from six a week to one every two weeks, parents obviously will not need to keep a written record of such a dramatic improvement.

Should a child with epilepsy carry an identification card or wear a badge such as those used by patients with diabetes?

It would probably be advisable for all individuals who have to take daily medications to prevent episodes during which they may lose consciousness to carry some form of identification, in the eventuality that one of these episodes should occur away from home or in strange surroundings. However, the great majority of older children and adolescents (and adults too) with epilepsy, object or have serious misgivings about carrying or wearing any kind of identification in the form of a card, bracelet, necklace, or similar device. The main reason given to justify this attitude is that the wearing of such devices will be a constant reminder to them and to others of a condition most of them are trying to forget and sometimes to hide. Because the use of these devices may be a source of additional emotional burden for older children and adolescents, we believe that in the great majority of cases it is up to the individual patient to decide whether or not to carry some type of identification.

We strongly believe, however, that in some epileptic children the use of some kind of identification *is* definitely indicated. Thus we strongly recommend the use of a readily apparent identification device by older children and teenagers with frequent or prolonged grand mal or psychomotor seizures, and by those in whom seizures are followed either by a prolonged state of impaired awareness or by unconsciousness.

Until recently most states had laws containing provisions for the "involuntary" sterilization of epileptics. Are there any social or medical indications for the "voluntary" sterilization of epileptics?

Dr. Samuel Livingston in his textbook *Comprehensive Management of Epilepsy in Infancy, Childhood and Adolescence** mentions two indications, one social, the other medical, for the voluntary sterilization of adult female epileptics. The social indication is that in which an epileptic woman who already has children "develops frequent and severe epileptic seizures which have been refractory to all available antiepileptic regimens." Dr. Livingston makes this recommendation "not because we feared that the patient would produce an epileptic offspring, but because we believed that there

* Samuel Livingston, *Comprehensive Management of Epilepsy in Infancy, Childhood and Adolescence* (Springfield, Illinois: Charles C. Thomas, 1972).

would be a great possibility that the afflicted individual would be unable to care for additional children." The medical indication proposed by Dr. Livingston is the case of "an epileptic female who suffered seizures during a previous pregnancy of such severity that they were a threat to her life. . . . We would recommend sterilization in such instances to prevent possible death to the patient during a subsequent pregnancy."

We agree entirely with Dr. Livingston's recommendations.

What about "voluntary" sterilization of older children or adolescents? Are there any reasons to sterilize a child with epilepsy?

On more than one occasion parents of epileptic children have asked us this question. In all instances, the child, usually a female, in addition to having epilepsy, was moderately retarded (IQ between 50 and 60), was thus not a suitable candidate for institutionalization, but, because of her low IQ, was not going to be able to live a completely independent life. I must admit from the outset that this is a sticky question and its answer is possibly a matter of opinion. There exist a number of personal, religious, social, as well as legal considerations which have to be considered in the making of such a drastic and irreversible decision.

Yet my personal opinion is that in many cases sterilization of older children or adolescents with epilepsy, who are also mentally retarded, should not only be entertained but is definitely indicated. Indeed, I must confess that my feelings on this problem approach downright dogmatism. Thus, whenever parents have requested my advice on this matter, I have not hesitated to recommend sterilization of mentally retarded female epileptics, especially when the affected child happens to be attractive. I believe it is difficult to find a valid reason to oppose the sterilization of a child who fulfills the above-mentioned criteria, and who is certainly a prime candidate for having an unwanted pregnancy.

Should infants with seizures be immunized for the common diseases of childhood at the same age as other infants?

During the past twenty-five years there has been a great deal of controversy among pediatricians regarding immunization of infants with seizures or of infants or young children with some sort of neurologic disorder. This controversy started in 1948 when Dr. R. K. Byers and Dr. F. C. Moll reported in the journal *Pediatrics* a group of fifteen children who had developed moderate to severe cerebral symptoms shortly after being immunized against whooping cough. Subsequent reports also emphasized that because of the possibility of cerebral complications children with any kind of neurological condition or epilepsy should not receive immunizations at the same age as normal infants. Based on these reports, in subsequent years many physicians throughout the country withheld immunizations against whooping cough to thousands of infants and young children with a history of seizures. Later studies, however, failed to prove that children with seizures or disorders affecting the nervous system are more prone than normal children to develop serious reactions to routine immunizations of early childhood. The *Report of the Committee on Infectious Diseases of the American Academy of Pediatrics* states in its 1974 edition:

Neurologic disorders in infants and children do not constitute a valid reason for deferring or withholding routine immunization. There is no clear-cut evidence that children with brain damage or convulsive disorders have a higher incidence of serious reactions from routine immunization procedures than do normal children. If there is no untoward reaction to any of the antigens, the recommended schedule for normal, healthy children is followed. If a central nervous system reaction occurs shortly after any dose of antigen,* defer immunization until the child reaches at least 1 year of age and evidence of active cerebral irritation has subsided. . . . Febrile reactions may be minimized by giving acetylsalicylic acid [aspirin] or acetaminophen [Tylenol], with or without phenobarbital in the appropriate dosage for age and weight, for 3 days following the immunization procedure.

Are there any environmental factors which can bring on seizures or increase their severity or their frequency?

Yes, but very few and they are of importance in only a very small number of epileptics. Over the years the importance of environmental influences of any kind as precipitating or aggravating factors of seizures has been greatly overemphasized. Public beliefs in this regard are difficult to explain. We often hear parents who wonder whether things that the child does or doesn't do, or something that they do or fail to do, or school or family situations, or temper tantrums, can bring on a seizure. Parents also often wonder about the influence on seizures of certain foods, vitamin deficiency, lack of sleep, or too much physical or mental exercise.

For unknown reasons most parents appear somewhat bewildered or amazed when their physicians tell them that in the vast majority of children with epilepsy there is very little that the child can do or not do to bring on a seizure. Frustrating situations and temper tantrums may precipitate a breath-holding spell, but practically never a true epileptic seizure. Also there is no scientific basis whatever to support the widespread belief among the general public that a poor intake of vitamins may cause or aggravate seizures. For one thing, epilepsy does not occur more frequently in countries where vitamin deficiency is prevalent in the general population.

---

* The name given to a substance which, when introduced into the body, causes the production of an antibody which will protect the individual from getting a disease such as diphtheria, whooping cough, tetanus, or poliomyelitis.

Furthermore, the ingestion of vitamins in excess of the daily body requirements has proved to have no influence on the frequency or severity of seizures. Although there is no medical proof that lack of sleep or physical exhaustion can produce a seizure in a person who is not an epileptic, it is possible that in some epileptic children these two factors may occasionally have some influence in precipitating a seizure.

Are there any situations during which seizures are more likely to occur?

Yes. Something is known, for example, about the influence of time of the day and changes in body functions in relation to the occurrence of seizures. Physicians have known for many years that sleep is as good a time as any to have seizures. They have also known for a long time that in some patients with epilepsy the electroencephalogram becomes abnormal only when the patient falls asleep. The same appears to be true of seizure occurrence. In many patients, seizures tend to occur only during periods of deep sleep about one to two hours after falling asleep, or shortly before awakening. The same applies to naps.

Why do some persons have seizures only or primarily during sleep?

Nobody knows for certain. It has been only during the past two decades that researchers have begun to investigate the great variety of changes taking place during sleep in different organs of the human body including the brain. Even though at least one-third of our lives is spent in sleep, it wasn't until the early 1950's that investigators began to work on this very fundamental biologic process. It soon became apparent that sleep was far from being just a state of total inactivity and comfortable rest. Nowadays it is well established that sleep is a complicated phenomenon which consists of a series of cyclic stages occurring at more or less predictable intervals throughout the night. One of these stages of sleep is characterized by rapid eye movements and is usually associated with dreams. During this stage the body temperature is elevated, the body metabolism is increased and the electrical rhythms recorded by the electroencephalograph are very similar to those seen when a person is awake. In contrast to this stage of rapid eye movements, there are three other stages during which the person falls progressively into deepening levels of sleep. The deeper stages are usually reached within the first two hours after falling asleep and again one to two hours before awakening. Physicians have known for a long time that these are the periods of sleep during which seizures may occur. It appears that as the depth of sleep increases the electrical rhythms of the brain become more and more synchronized, thus predisposing susceptible individuals to the development of seizures. As I mentioned in Chapter 1, a high degree of synchronized activity, good as it may be for a battalion or a kindergarten class, is simply not good for the human brain.

Can menstrual periods influence the occurrence of seizures in patients with epilepsy?

Definitely. Some females have seizures more frequently or only at a particular time of their menstrual cycle. When this happens, it is usually during the days preceding menstruation or during the first or second day after the onset of the menstrual flow. Moreover, it is not too uncommon for girls whose seizures have been under control for several years to have a recurrence at the onset of puberty. Occasionally a girl whose seizures have never been completely under control may experience more frequent or more severe convulsions after the onset of menstruation.

Seizures which occur primarily at a certain time in the

menstrual cycle are often difficult to control. Through the years physicians have resorted to special therapeutic regimens, such as increasing the amount of anticonvulsant drugs for a few days prior to the time when seizures are expected to occur during the menstrual cycle; restricting fluid and salt for a couple of days prior to and during the period of menstrual flow; or giving a diuretic to promote the elimination by the kidneys of accumulated fluid. Unfortunately, in a large number of females none of these measures is successful in controlling seizures. It can be of little consolation for the adolescent girl with intractable menstrual seizures to know that this type of attack frequently ceases spontaneously at the time of menopause! On the basis of this empirical observation some physicians have recommended the use of female hormones to induce an artificial menopause. This type of treatment, however, has by no means proved to be consistently successful. And not only that. Frequently the side effects of hormonal treatment can produce more incapacitating symptoms than the seizures.

The exact mechanism by which menstruation affects the brain of only some female epileptics is unknown. We also know little about the influence on the brain of the many hormonal changes taking place during the menstrual cycle. It is possible that excessive retention of water may play an important role.

What about other illnesses or high fever?

Sudden elevations of temperature due to infections of any kind (usually a throat or ear infection) can produce grand mal seizures in children less than five years of age. If the seizures occur only in association with febrile illnesses and are of short duration, they are called febrile seizures. As noted in Chapter 1, the great majority of children with febrile seizures are not truly epileptics: nine out of ten spontaneously outgrow this tendency to convulse during diseases associated with fever by the age of five years and never again will experience another seizure (see also page 20). In addition to febrile seizures of early childhood, fever due to just about any illness can also precipitate seizures in children with other types of seizures. It is not at all unusual to see children, for example, whose seizures are well controlled with drug treatment except when they develop an infection of some kind.

What else can bring on a seizure?

The most important and dangerous precipitating factor of seizures in patients with epilepsy is the abrupt withdrawal of anticonvulsant medications. Sudden withdrawal of medications can occur for a variety of reasons. Many well-motivated parents somehow convince themselves that because their child has been seizure-free for six or twelve months he no longer needs to take medication. On other occasions an older child may on his own stop taking the medication without his parents' knowledge. It is our feeling that in most of these cases the only reason for stopping treatment without previously consulting the treating physician is the fear that prolonged treatment with anticonvulsants may slow down the mental development of the child or interfere with his ability to learn in school. In other cases it is due to lack of precise instructions from physicians, or to parents' failure to understand these instructions, regarding the length of time that a child with epilepsy should receive anticonvulsant therapy. Sometimes the obvious can also happen. Parents simply run out of medicines during a weekend and the child may thus skip three, four, or more doses until a new prescription is filled. In other instances, parents may just forget to give the child his medicine.

Sudden withdrawal of anticonvulsants is not only the best way to bring on a seizure, it is also the most common cause of status epilepticus. It cannot be stressed enough then that anticonvulsant treatment should be given on a *continuous*, daily basis. We know we are saying what is obvious, but the only safe way to avoid running out of medications is to refill prescriptions at least one or two weeks before the bottle is completely empty. It is not uncommon for physicians to receive phone calls from parents during a weekend and hear that "Johnny just ran out of medicine." Remember that it is always better to prevent than to cure. In many states physicians cannot "write" prescriptions over the phone and in most areas of the country pharmacists are not authorized to refill prescriptions for more than six months without a new "verbal" or written prescription from the treating physician. Last but not least, do not forget that you may be unable to reach your pediatrician or your family physician at the time Johnny took the last tablet left in the bottle.

All these considerations serve to point out the urgent need of having available at all times a good supply of anticonvulsants. Even though I know you couldn't possibly have already forgotten what I have just said I am going to repeat it anyhow. If anticonvulsants are suddenly withdrawn one of three things may happen to your child: (1) nothing, (2) his seizures may recur after a prolonged period of remission while taking medicines, or (3) he may go into a series of grand mal seizures known as status epilepticus which is not only a potentially dangerous situation in terms of brain damage; it may also end fatally.

What else can precipitate seizures?

Overbreathing or hyperventilation is known to be an excellent precipitating factor of petit mal attacks. Rarely, hyperventilation may also induce or bring on other types of seizures. While a person hyperventilates there is an excessive loss of a gas called carbon dioxide (CO_2) which is normally exchanged for oxygen (O_2) during respiration. The excessive loss of CO_2 leads to a disturbance in the equilibrium of these gases normally present in the blood and body tissues, including the brain. In everyday life, however, hyperventilation due to physical exertion or other reasons is not of the magnitude needed to precipitate any type of seizure.

Occasionally one sees a child whose seizures are brought on by sudden changes in the intensity of natural or artificial light. Seizures may occur, for example, if the child is suddenly exposed to bright sunlight when coming out of the house. The flickering lights from a defective television set may also have the same effect. In rare instances other environmental stimuli, such as music or reading, may also precipitate a seizure.

What types of seizures are brought on by sudden changes in light or by music or reading?

Seizures brought on by exposure to bright or flickering lights, or by other environmental stimuli such as music or reading, are almost always of the minor motor type. On rare occasions, grand mal seizures may also occur. When one of these children is exposed to one of the previously mentioned stimuli, he may lose consciousness for two or three seconds, may fall abruptly to the ground and get up immediately, or may repeatedly and purposelessly flutter his eyelids for a couple of seconds.

Seizures which are precipitated by sudden exposure to bright or flickering lights are particularly resistant to treatment with anticonvulsant drugs. It has been suggested that the wearing of deeply-tinted blue glasses or of a wide-brimmed "Greta Garbo" type hat during summer months may be useful in preventing seizures in some of these children. It is obvious that continuous avoidance of the precipitating factor (light, music, reading) is for all practical purposes impossible.

Can drugs precipitate a seizure in an epileptic child?

A number of drugs have been incriminated in the past as possible precipitators of seizures. Among these, the best-documented ones are phenothiazine derivatives. The phenothiazine drugs (Thorazine, Compazine) are very widely used in the practice of medicine. They are used primarily in the treatment of vomiting, and in the treatment of psychiatric disorders. As noted in Chapter 1, a convulsion occurs when a group of brain cells produces a large number of highly synchronized electrical discharges. It has been postulated that the mechanism of action of phenothiazine drugs in causing seizures is "the activation of a preexisting epileptic predisposition or lesser resistance to seizures by suppressing the desynchronizing effects of sensory stimuli from the environment on the electrical discharges of the brain." This complicated and pompous sentence means simply that the stimuli from the environment that reach the brain through our senses produce a state of more or less constant desynchronization of brain-wave rhythms. When for some reason, such as the administration of phenothiazine or other drugs, this desynchronizing influence on the brain is suppressed, the result may be an excessive amount of synchronization of brain-wave rhythms, which may produce a seizure in an individual with a lesser resistance to seizures.

Are there certain things which a child with seizures should not be allowed to do?

In my experience, not too many parents ask this question. It would seem that this is one question which they are either afraid to ask or which they have themselves already answered. I, as well as most physicians who treat children with seizures, have the distinct impression that the youngster with epilepsy is too often an overprotected child whose physical activities are curtailed well beyond reasonable limits.

I believe that there are very few things that a child whose seizures are under control should not be allowed to do. Common sense, of course, indicates that exposure to dangerous situations such as tree climbing, playing basketball on top of the roof, or bicycle riding in heavy traffic should be discouraged.

What about bicycle riding, baseball, basketball, and especially football?

Well, and what about walking, running, eating, and crossing the street? Cannot all of these activities in many ways also represent hazardous situations at the time of a seizure? Of course they can. And they can be dangerous not only for the child who has seizures, but also for just about anybody. We have to face the fact that as long as a person is alive there is really no place where he can be entirely safe at all times. If a child with epilepsy is to have any chance at all of developing as an emotionally mature individual, he should live as normal a life as possible. There are certain things which just about everybody should be allowed to do. In this regard we should remember that most adults, at least in this country, have occasion to drive a car every single day of their lives. Who can deny then that for at least one hour a day all of us are more or less in constant and serious danger? There is little need to make reference to people such as construction workers, policemen, or firemen, whose jobs include additional built-in dangers. Whether we like it or not, all of us are forced to take hundreds of chances every single day of our lives.

The only sensible answer to a question like this is a sensible compromise between the dangers involved in the performance of a certain activity and the disadvantages of going through life without the benefit of it. (See also page 193 in regard to competitive athletics and the epileptic child.)

Do children with epilepsy suffer more frequent or more serious injuries than other children?

No. It seems only reasonable to suspect that children with epilepsy have to suffer more frequent or more serious injuries than other children. But on the basis of our experience with hundreds of patients, as well as the observations made by other physicians who have treated thousands of epileptic children, we can say that, with the exception of patients with myoclonic seizures, the incidence of bodily injuries is not higher in patients with epilepsy than in the general population. And not only that. I am fully convinced that epileptic children suffer less-frequent and less-serious injuries or accidents than other children. The only reason I can find to explain this is that, irrespective of how well controlled their seizures may be, epileptics seem to be more careful about the risks of everyday life, and most of them, especially adolescents, are also more careful than their peers in exposing themselves to needlessly dangerous situations.

What can be done to prevent injuries in a child with myoclonic seizures?

First, what is obvious: the child should receive appropriate anticonvulsant treatment. Second, if his seizures are not under control, buy him something to protect his head. As mentioned in Chapter 1, myoclonic seizures are characterized by a sudden flexion jerk of the head, the extremities, or the entire body. If the muscle jerk is severe the child falls to the ground as violently as if somebody had thrown him down. Consequently, as long as a child with myoclonic seizures has frequent attacks, I strongly urge his parents to have the child wear a leather helmet or a similar protective device while he is up and around. Parents often wonder if it isn't awkward or embarrassing for a child to wear a helmet. As a rule it isn't. We should remember that myoclonic seizures occur primarily in young children. And children at this age are not terribly self-conscious about things like wearing a helmet in front of other people. Moreover, it doesn't take these children very long to realize that this "inconvenience" is a far better deal than going to the emergency room of a hospital every two weeks to get stitches for a chin or a scalp laceration.

What about special indications or restrictions in food, beverages, exercise, or sleep?

In regard to all these items I can say that moderation is the only rule. Obesity is of course always undesirable; it is from a medical standpoint a disease, and certainly in the long run much more serious than epilepsy. Since this is a manual primarily for parents of children with seizures I do not have to point out that alcoholic beverages, although effective sedatives, do not have anticonvulsant properties. Not only that; it is the opinion of internists and adult neurologists that the excessive intake of alcoholic beverages appears to increase the frequency and severity of just about any type of seizure. Similarly there is little need to emphasize that physical exhaustion should be avoided in health as well as in disease. On the other hand, physical exercise, within the limits of individual tolerance, should be encouraged. It seems that inactivity is harmful to the epileptic child and that physical exercise as well as a busy mind are good seizure deterrents.

By the same token there is little need to underscore the fact that everybody needs to have an adequate number of hours of sleep and rest. Of course these needs vary considerably from one individual to another. Any person, child or adult, and whether healthy or sick, should only sleep as many hours as he needs. Forcing an epileptic child to sleep or rest more than he actually needs will be of no help to him.

If a child has seizures only during the nighttime, should he sleep in his parent's bedroom? Or should one of the parents sleep in his bedroom?

Some children with epilepsy have seizures only during the night while they are asleep. They represent, however, a relatively small percentage of all epileptic children. A much larger group of children have diurnal (daytime) as well as nocturnal (nighttime) seizures.

We have known a number of well-motivated parents who for years have made their epileptic child sleep in their bedroom even though his seizures were well controlled with anticonvulsant medication. We believe that this custom is in the great majority of cases not only entirely unjustified but also a bit nonsensical. It seems reasonable that if a child has grand mal seizures only while asleep, one of the parents may wish to sleep in the child's bedroom until his seizures are controlled by anticonvulsant medications. The primary objective of this policy is, of course, to assess the efficacy of anticonvulsant treatment. Parents ought to realize, however, that with the exception of grand mal seizures all other forms of epilepsy can go unrecognized even if both parents and the child are sleeping in one bed. As long as the daytime attacks of a child who has both diurnal and nocturnal seizures are well controlled, there is no reason to believe that the same is not true of seizures which occur during the night. Why overprotect your child by making him feel that he needs you even when he really doesn't?

10. The Epileptic Child and Society

When a child with seizures grows up, will he be able to get married and if he does so, will he be able to have children?

Until recently several states had laws which forbade epileptics to marry. This as well as other archaic state laws were passed at a time when epilepsy was considered to be an incurable disease which eventually led to insanity. At the present time there is absolutely no medical reason to support the belief that a person with epilepsy should not marry and, if he gets married, that he shouldn't have children. The only exception to this rule is probably the epileptic of average intelligence who, because of very frequent attacks which cannot be controlled with anticonvulsants, will not be capable of supporting a family.

Can a teen-ager with epilepsy obtain a driver's license?

Yes. Today teen-agers with epilepsy are able to obtain licenses to drive motor vehicles in all fifty states. The only prerequisite is a medical certificate stating that his seizures have been under control for a reasonable period of time, and that, in the opinion of a physician experienced in the treatment of seizures, the patient will make a reasonable driving risk. The length of a "reasonable period of time" varies in

178

different states from six months to three years. In a few states driver's licenses are granted on the basis of the frequency of a patient's seizures, on the recommendations of the treating physician, and sometimes only after the state medical review board has gone over a particular case.

American adolescents look forward to their sixteenth birthday with a great deal of anticipation. This is the age at which most states will grant a teen-ager a license to drive a motor vehicle. If a child is still having seizures when he reaches the age of fourteen or fifteen, he should be told that in all probability he will not be granted a driver's license at sixteen and that he will have to wait one, two, or more years before he may be able to obtain one. In our experience the emotional trauma that goes along with the inability to obtain a driver's license at the expected age is either lessened or completely eliminated if an epileptic child is told about it in advance and is thus prepared to cope with what for most of them is doubtless a serious social handicap.

Are state laws still particularly hard on people with epilepsy?

No, they are not. But significant changes in many obsolete state laws which made life extremely hard for the epileptic did not take place until recent years. In more than one respect things have not always been easy for epileptics. Until 1957, seventeen states prohibited epileptics from marrying and nineteen states had laws concerning involuntary sterilization of epileptics. Until very recently, in at least one state applications for marriage licenses included a question as to whether the applicant was "not an idiot, epileptic or common drunkard." Up to 1968 U. S. immigration laws prohibited the entrance to this country of people with a history of seizures—and not only for those who wished to reside permanently in this country, but also for those who wanted to come for medical diagnosis and treatment. Until 1957, less than half of the states were willing to grant a driver's license to persons who had had seizures in the past, and when a license was given, it was always under very special circumstances. In 1959 Wisconsin became the first state to grant driver's licenses to epileptics whose seizures had been under control for two years. It is ironic that during the next ten years the accident records of epileptics in Wisconsin was, on the average, four times better than that of other drivers.

By the same token, until recent years it was practically impossible for a person with a history of seizures to obtain liability insurance of any kind.

How difficult is it for the epileptic nowadays to get life or other types of insurance?

Not too difficult, but he may go broke in the process! In regard to life insurance, the policy of one of the largest United States insurance companies is as follows:

Of the various forms of epilepsy grand mal is the more serious. . . . Applicants under age 15, those with more than eight seizures per year or where attacks are becoming frequent and severe, are not offered life insurance. This is also true for those whose epilepsy is caused by some known chronic brain disorder. Other cases, adequately controlled by medication, are placed in impairment classes depending upon the interval since the last seizure. Especially favorable cases with no seizure for ten years may be taken Standard. DP [disability payment or waiver of premium] is not offered. Petit mal is considered to be a more benign condition than grand mal, but they often coexist and childhood petit mal may develop into grand mal. Applicants under age 5 are not considered. Otherwise, an individual in good health and under good control is considered moderately impaired for at least two years following his last seizure. Thereafter, more favorable ratings are offered and some select cases are accepted Standard after five years. DP is not available.

In respect to health and disability insurance the same company states:

Applicants under age 19 and those whose attacks commence within five years of application or who experience more than five attacks per year, will not be considered. Other cases are considered moderately to severely impaired for an indefinite period (grand mal) or for at least five years (petit mal) for all types of insurance.

In selected cases insurance companies are able to offer automobile insurance to epileptics at standard premiums. This is, however, the rare exception. Higher premiums are still paid by the great majority of people with a history of seizures, even by those who have not had an attack for a number of years. We believe that this is an unfair as well as an unwise policy on the part of insurance companies. As long as the division of motor vehicles of a particular state considers a person with epilepsy a reasonable driving risk, and is willing to grant him a license to drive a motor vehicle, we see no valid reason for insurance companies to discriminate against a person with a history of epilepsy. In the long run this type of policy can lead only to an increase in the number of people who will conceal having had seizures in the past.

These general guidelines pretty well summarize current policies of United States insurance companies with regard to the insurability of people with epilepsy. The general rule is consideration on an individual basis. And as can be expected, this "consideration" is in most cases a lopsided affair, the insurance company taking more than the necessary and fair precautions to protect its interests.

Is an epileptic teen-ager liable for harm inflicted on another person as a result of a seizure occurring while driving a car?

The legal aspects of epilepsy have been extensively reviewed by R. L. Barrow and H. D. Fabing in their book *Epilepsy and the Law*. In regard to the civil liability of an epileptic who has a seizure while driving a motor vehicle, they state:

The operative principles governing civil liability of an epileptic automobile driver are as follows. If the epileptic has obtained a license under a procedure which took his condition into account ... is following the regimen of treatment prescribed by his doctor, and is cooperating with his doctor in reporting any change of condition which relates to his ability to drive safely, he is not liable for civil negligence in the event that a seizure should occur. The state's licensing authority has evaluated, with the aid of the applicant's doctor, the ability of the epileptic to operate a motor vehicle with reasonable safety and has approved him as a reasonable driving risk. He is duly licensed to drive an automobile on the public highways. Under the circumstances stated, the epileptic has taken the precautions which he is under a duty to exercise. If under all these circumstances, a seizure and resulting injury to another person should occur, the epileptic would not be civilly liable for negligence, whether a person outside the epileptic's automobile or a passenger is injured.

On the other hand, the epileptic would be civilly liable for negligence to a person other than a guest passenger in the event that a seizure occurs and there is resulting loss of control of the automobile and injury, under the following circumstances: the epileptic knows that he is subject to seizures and conceals the condition when applying for a license or, if having obtained a license after disclosure and evaluation of his ability to drive safely, the seizures recur and the epileptic conceals this information from his doctor and the licensing authority. This is because the epileptic, under the circumstances specified, reasonably should have known that a seizure might occur while he was driving and that, in the event of a seizure, other users of the highway might be injured or killed. It is not clear whether civil liability, under the circumstances outlined, would extend to a passenger in the epileptic's automobile in view of the guest statute standard of reckless operation of the motor vehicle. Certainty as to the law on this point must await the outcome of future cases.

Is an epileptic responsible for acts of violence committed during the course of a seizure?

The above mentioned authors answer this question as follows:

Among those conditions which may be considered as a possible defense, to an indictment of crime, on the ground of insanity is epilepsy. When an epileptic is charged with a crime of violence—particularly if it is a cause célèbre such as the recent trial of Jack Ruby on the charge of murdering the assassin of President Kennedy—the public may gain the impression that a common characteristic of epilepsy is a tendency to commit acts of violence. Most epileptics are normal people except during a seizure and the seizure usually manifests itself in a condition which renders the epileptic incapable of inflicting harm on others. There is no evidence that the incidence of commission of unlawful acts is higher among epileptics than among the population as a whole. However, a few epileptics may experience psychomotor seizures characterized by automatism, in which state an act of violence may occur. If an unlawful act is committed by an epileptic while in a state of automatism, the question arises as to whether the epileptic is criminally responsible for his act. . . .

In the present state of the law, generally automatism as a result of psychomotor seizures is a valid defense to a charge of crime for committing an unlawful act while unconscious. The dearth of cases using this defense is explained by two factors. One is the problem of proof. If a person is conscious immediately prior to commission of an unlawful act and conscious immediately after commission of the unlawful act, the prosecutor may satisfy the jury that the particular violent act occurred during a conscious period rather than during a psychomotor seizure involving unconsciousness and automatism. The other factor is that incidence of psychomotor epilepsy is rare and the ordinary epileptic does not commit acts of violence during a seizure and would have no reason to use the insanity defense on the basis of epilepsy.

Dr. Samuel Livingston of the Johns Hopkins Hospital, on the basis of more than thirty years of experience with epileptics of all ages, says in regard to criminal acts committed by epileptics:

We have not found evidence of a higher rate of criminal activity among epileptics than among nonepileptics. On the basis of thirty-five years' contact with the course of living of approximately twenty thousand epileptic patients on every social level, we can state positively that the incidence of crimes committed by these patients was no greater than—even showed no difference from—that in a similar number of nonepileptics.

We would not question the fact than an epileptic might kill, not because he has epilepsy, but because he is a human being. However, we would like to state emphatically that the violation of the Sixth Commandment is not indigenous to epilepsy and that an epileptic is no more a potential murderer than the so-called normal individual.*

Do these changes in state laws mean that the attitude of the general public toward the person with epilepsy has radically changed in the last two decades?

No, it does not. But it *is* changing, slowly. Although during the past twenty years important changes have taken place in many of the previously mentioned areas, when it comes to opportunities for employment, for example, the epileptic is today still the subject of discrimination.

A number of large industrial companies have long recognized that as a rule the physically handicapped person makes a very good employee. It is ironic then that thousands of epileptics whose seizures are well controlled are still the subject of discrimination even though they are not truly physically handicapped individuals. It is about time for society at large and for employers in particular to abandon these obso-

* William G. Lennox, "Therapeutics of Epilepsy," *Therapeutic Notes* 61, *Childhood and Adolescence* (Springfield, Illinois: Charles C. Thomas, 1972), p. 551.

lete, discriminatory policies and to realize that valid reasons no longer exist to stick to the erroneous belief that the epileptic is a person incapable of leading a normal and productive life. The general public should also become aware that the epileptic suffers from a chronic disorder which is in no way different from many other chronic illnesses which affect man, such as diabetes, high blood pressure, or duodenal ulcer.

Why, then, is the epileptic the object of discrimination? Why do so many people still today seem to think of him almost as if he were a being from a different species?

For several reasons. First of all, we have to realize that for most people it is not easy to get rid of deeply rooted biases and prejudices. It might be easier to understand this type of reaction if we remember that the epileptic has been stigmatized for more than two thousand years. Ancient Greeks were already referring to epilepsy as the "falling sickness" and also as the "sacred disease." Its very name seemed to carry the implication that there was something weird about it; something out of the ordinary; something which in a way did not seem to belong to this world. The word "epilepsy," in Greek meaning "to seize upon," meant that during an epileptic attack the person was suddenly possessed by supernatural forces. We must also remember that as recently as forty years ago the medical profession knew very little about epilepsy and that up to that time the disorder was still a condition surrounded by mystery and superstition.

All the previously mentioned state laws, which in many ways officially stigmatized the epileptic and made him a second-class citizen, were passed during the latter part of the nineteenth century at a time when epilepsy was still considered to be a strange and incurable condition which often led to progressive mental deterioration—and at a time when the children of such individuals were considered likely to inherit the disease. Doubtless the increasing medical knowl-

edge of the past thirty years as well as the development of
effective drugs for the treatment of epilepsy have in no small
measure contributed to clarify the true nature of the condition, the few, if any, limitations imposed upon people who
have the disorder, and the relative ease with which seizures
can be brought under control with appropriate drug treatment. But we must realize that it is not easy to eradicate
prejudices which have been passed on for so many years from
one generation to the next.

In the final analysis we can say that the only reason for the
persistence of these unfair attitudes toward the epileptic has
been nothing but a very long period of ignorance on the part
of the general public and physicians alike regarding the true
nature, outlook, and genetic implications of epilepsy. There
can be little doubt that as more people become aware of what
epilepsy really is these prejudices will disappear altogether.
As pointed out by Dr. William Lennox,* in spite of the
miraculous advances made in the drug treatment of epilepsy
during the past twenty years,

Social therapy has not paralleled medical advance. Epilepsy
lacks the widespread public interest and support accorded certain
other less hopeful disorders of the nervous system. Hippocrates,
if he returned, would be amazed and incredulous at [the] sight of
the electroencephalograph, the excision of damaged portions of
brains, and the truly miraculous effect of anticonvulsant drugs.
But he might well consider us backward in social treatment. The
Greeks regarded the epileptic as god-possessed, surely a position
of respect, and accorded to him the rights of education and employment, rights often denied now.

**Isn't it difficult to believe that until forty years ago physicians
knew very little about epilepsy?**

No, it is not. Forty years ago physicians also knew very
little about a great many other medical problems. Worse yet,

* William G. Lennox, "Therapeutics of Epilepsy," *Therapeutic Notes* 61,
no. 5 (May 1954):136.

even today misconceptions and sometimes downright erroneous concepts about epilepsy exist not only among practicing physicians, but also among medical writers of books for the layman. Dr. Paul Kühne, for example, in his *Home Medical Encyclopedia** (revised edition), a book available in bookshops and wherever paperbacks are sold in the United States, ignores everything medical science has learned about epilepsy during the past half century, and repeats ideas which enjoyed popularity during the eighteenth and nineteenth centuries.

In Dr. Kühne's "encyclopedia" the following statements can be found: "epileptics are highly irritable and may fly into a rage over trivialities" . . . "epilepsy often occurs with schizophrenia" . . . "a typical mental characteristic [of the epileptic] is the fact that their outlook remains immature. In everything they do they try to assert themselves by outdoing others rather than by achieving a definite aim." . . . "These attacks themselves may disappear temporarily or permanently or be replaced by minor mental symptoms, i.e. a sudden fit of complete absent-mindedness, which occurs with lightning swiftness and is only temporary, or an inexplicable and strange mood of depression, which is also of short duration" . . . "in treating epilepsy one tries to suppress the patient's excitement and with it the attacks by means of sedatives." None of these statements could be further from the truth.

As we will see in Chapter 12 there is not and there has never been such a thing as a stereotyped epileptic personality. The epileptic like any other individual can, according to his own unique personality and under different circumstances, fly into just about anything. Attacks of rage over trivialities are no more common in epileptics than in so-called "normal" people. Dr. Kühne's pronouncement on the relationship between epilepsy and schizophrenia is not a misconception but a flagrant mistake, which unfortunately is bound to inflict a

* Paul Kühne, *Home Medical Encyclopedia*, trans. Geon Cunningham (Greenwich, Conn.: Fawcett, 1960).

great deal of unnecessary emotional damage on adult epileptics as well as on parents of children with epilepsy. For many years psychiatrists have known that the incidence of schizophrenia in people with epilepsy is considerably *less* than in the general population. Dr. Lothar Kalinowsky states in Alfred Freedman and Harold Kaplan's *Comprehensive Textbook of Psychiatry* in regard to the history and rationale of convulsive therapy in the treatment of patients with schizophrenia: "It had been noted for a long time by mental hospital physicians that patients would suddenly lose their symptoms when they had a spontaneous convulsion, no matter what caused it. The second line of reasoning was based on various statistics showing that epilepsy and schizophrenia hardly ever occurred in the same patient." Moreover, it is well known that epileptics do not share common psychological characteristics of any kind. In this regard, Dr. Kühne ignores the fundamental concepts that epilepsy is not a single disease, but is only a symptom of intermittent, abnormal electrical brain discharges due to a variety of causes. It is only obvious that, since no two epileptics are alike, they cannot possibly have in common any special mental or psychologic characteristics.

The reader needs only to recall what we have already said in Chapter 1 regarding the many different forms that epileptic attacks may take to realize that, when Dr. Kühne writes about inexplicable short-lasting episodes of "absentmindedness," he is really referring to "nonshaking" epileptic attacks rather than to any unusual psychologic or emotional phenomena.

In Chapter 5 we discussed in some detail several aspects of the drug, dietary, and surgical treatment of epilepsy. Regrettably, Dr. Kühne's statement about the treatment of seizures ignores completely the very existence of specific drugs for the treatment of epilepsy.

11. Epilepsy and the School Child

What can a teacher do should an attack occur in school?

During the attack, not as much as he would like to stop it. After the attack is over, he may end up doing much less than what he can and should do. See page 157 for description of measures that can be taken to help a child during a grand mal seizure.

Should a child be sent home from school after a seizure?

It all depends on the individual. If the child is back to normal immediately after the attack, there is really little reason to send him home.

What if a child has more than one seizure in a single day?

If the seizures are mild, or are of the petit mal or minor motor types, again there is little justification to send the child home. Decisions in this respect, however, should be highly individualized. If the child is drowsy or sleepy after a seizure, or if he should show any other after-effects, he should be *taken* home. Teachers should notify the parents of such an occurrence, especially if this has been the child's first seizure. Teachers as well as parents should keep mental track of the approximate frequency and nature of the seizures so that they can pass on this information to the physician.

Is there anything that the teacher can do after the attack is over?

Yes. Actually, after the seizure is over is when the teacher's job really begins. Not infrequently it ends even before it gets started, certainly a most unfortunate situation.

If at all possible the teacher should remain as calm as he can during and after an attack. Under the circumstances, this may be easier to say than to do. He should reassure the rest of his pupils that the world is not coming to an end and that what they have just seen is called a seizure; that their classmate once in a while has attacks just like the one they saw; that the attacks are not dangerous; and that he will be back to his normal self in a matter of a few minutes. If the children are old enough to understand, the teacher can give them a brief explanation of epilepsy, and can let them know that persons with this disorder need to take medicines in the form of a tablet or a capsule one or more times daily to prevent the recurrence of attacks.

It seems only fair that teachers as well as school nurses should be spared the unpleasant surprise of a child's first grand mal convulsion in school. If a child has epilepsy, they should be notified in advance by parents or physicians that he may very well have an attack in school. This way they will be in a better position to help the child during the course of a grand mal seizure, and unquestionably they will be more likely to remain calm and composed during the episode, and thus avoid becoming a cause of unjustified alarm for the rest of the pupils.

Following a seizure in school, or at home, the child should be treated as if nothing of great importance has taken place. In school as well as at home the child should be treated like any other child. He should not only be allowed but also encouraged to participate in school activities just as the rest of his classmates do.

Is it true that some public schools still refuse enrollment of children with epilepsy?

Yes, but the problem is not as widespread or as serious as it used to be. Some school officials still refuse to take or are reluctant to accept a child with epilepsy, even though his seizures may have been under satisfactory control for years. Arguments given in support of this policy are things such as the following: an epileptic child may get badly hurt during a seizure, a convulsion in the classroom may be disturbing or emotionally upsetting for the rest of the pupils, some parents don't want their children to be in the same classroom as a child with epilepsy, and so forth. It is quite obvious that all these reasons are unfounded.

There is no reason for teachers and school officials to be afraid of suits in case of injuries sustained as a result of an epileptic attack. If any questions in this respect should arise, parents can be asked to sign a release-of-responsibility form for injuries incurred during the course of a seizure. We said earlier that children with epilepsy do not get hurt more often and do not suffer more serious injuries than other children. The occasion of a seizure in the classroom can certainly be used by the teacher to the advantage of the education of the rest of his or her pupils. The teacher may be in a position to help them to understand better the true facts about a very common disorder, eliminate the fear the sight of a seizure may have generated and thus enable them to react in a more sympathetic and realistic way toward their classmate's ailment. A short explanation that a seizure is no more serious than a bad chest cold and something over which the child has no control will usually satisfy the curiosity of young children. Older pupils can be given a more detailed description of the problem.

Teachers and parents alike ought to remember that children cannot and should not be isolated from the unpleasant aspects of life. Furthermore, the teacher's attitude toward the epileptic child can greatly help him to avoid becoming socially isolated, and being the object of teasing and taunting by his classmates. Once a child knows that epilepsy is a disorder which is not "catching," he can begin to feel empathy for his affected classmate. Finally, parents who still complain about having a child with epilepsy in the same classroom as their own child will almost always change their minds when they learn or are told the facts about the disorder, especially if they obtain this information from their own child.

What is, in general, the attitude of teachers toward children with epilepsy?

The attitude of teachers toward epileptic children has changed a great deal during the past two decades. Not too many years ago, a study of teachers' knowledge of epilepsy and their personal reactions toward children with seizures revealed several interesting although disappointing findings. To begin with, epilepsy was found to be a much more common problem among school children than had been previously suspected. Misconceptions about the nature of the condition and the epileptic child in general were also common. The amount of information that teachers had about epilepsy was, more often than not, scanty. And it was found that the way teachers reacted to having a child with epilepsy in their classroom was largely determined by personal biases and emotional factors rather than by a clear understanding of the problem. As noted above, the attitude of teachers as well as that of other professionals involved in the care or education of children has changed considerably during the past twenty years. We believe that these changes have been due in no small measure to the unremitting efforts of a number of national and local organizations like the Epilepsy Foundation of America, which have fought, and partially won in a fairly short period of time, the battle against the ignorance and prejudice surrounding epilepsy.

Should a child with epilepsy participate in competitive school athletics?

A Committee on Children with Handicaps states in its report* of October, 1968, "The Epileptic Child and Competitive School Athletics":

In children with epilepsy, as in children with any chronic disorder, it is important that the patient and his family recognize early during the course of the disease that certain adjustments in the daily routine may need to be made. . . . However, from a quantitative [number] point of view, the major problem is the group of children with seizures of unknown etiology [cause] or idiopathic epilepsy. . . . An individual subject to frequent recurrences of such major seizures, despite competent medical management, may or may not be a candidate for competitive athletics. . . . Between the two extremes of petit mal and grand mal there is a spectrum of seizure states [types], the nature and severity of which require that each child receive highly individual consideration in the matter of his daily activity. . . . Both physical and mental activities seem to be seizure deterrents. Experience has shown that many epileptic patients have fewer seizures when they are active compared to when they are idle or at rest. . . . This has led to the general recommendation that most epileptic children should engage in all physical activities which do not impose a significant risk of injury to themselves or others. The majority of epileptic children participate in physical activities at school and in athletics with minimal difficulty; some epileptic children excel in athletics. Providing the epilepsy is under satisfactory control, many school systems make little distinction between epileptic and nonepileptic children in their participation in athletic programs. . . . One unresolved question is the potential exacerbation of preexisting organic pathology; but, if such events actually occur,

* Committee on Children with Handicaps, "The Epileptic Child and Competitive School Athletics," *Pediatrics* 42 (1968):700.

they are probably quite rare. Evidence is meager that closed head injuries resulting from body contact sports aggravate a preexisting epileptic disorder.

In regard to body contact sports the committee states:

If there is more than an occasional seizure, sports involving body contact should be considered on the basis of individual evaluation. . . . Individualization based on clinical history must be the rule in all cases.

In regard to gymnastics the committee states:

General agreement exists that epileptics should not perform athletic activities where a fall would result if a seizure were experienced without warning. These would include rope climbing, gymnastics involving parallel bars, trampolines, and so forth. Individual consideration remains the basic determinant.

In regard to swimming the committee states:

Most authorities believe that the epileptic patient should be allowed to participate in swimming activities with the understanding that he, like all other children, should always be under supervision. Accordingly, as with all children, competitive underwater swimming should be discouraged.

The committee also states:

The responsibility for weighing the risks involved in athletic participation should be considered by the parent, the physician, and the child. Such risks should be weighed against the psychological trauma resulting from unnecessarily restricting physical activities. . . . To the degree appropriate to the age and judgment of the child, his own wishes must be considered. . . . He must realize that there is a calculated risk of injury and be prepared to impose voluntary restrictions on himself, depending on the nature and frequency of his convulsions.

The committee concludes its report by saying that "recommendations should be highly individualized, taking into account a given child's seizure history."

A somewhat different view is expressed by a report of the American Medical Association Committee on the Medical Aspects of Sports and the Committee on Exercise and Physical Fitness entitled "Convulsive Disorders and Participation in Sports and Physical Education," also published in 1968, in the *Journal of the American Medical Association.** This committee offers the following recommendations:

Today it is generally accepted by both physicians and educators that young people with convulsive disorders, once the seizures are under reasonable control, should be encouraged to lead as normal and active a life as possible. This applies to participation in sports as well as to other types of physical activity. . . . Each situation is an individual one and cannot be classified under specified categories to which general rules apply. Therefore, in each instance there should be a definitive diagnosis, a careful health history review of the patient, and thoughtful planning of the medical and supporting management required. As a part of such management, a judgment should be made with respect to the individual's ability to participate without undue risk to either himself or his teammates. Three decisive factors in arriving at a reliable judgment on this matter are (1) whether good control of his condition is maintained by medication, (2) whether the extent and intensity of participation pose a significant threat to his physicial condition, and (3) whether the patient is cooperative and in control of any impulsiveness. . . . When this judgment favors participation in sports, the athlete, the parents and the athletic supervisory personnel should thoroughly understand the risks involved, the preventive measures to be taken and the values to be derived from competition in suitable sports. . . . When all the factors involved have been considered and properly evaluated, the youth concerned

* American Medical Association Committee on the Medical Aspects of Sports and the Committee on Exercise and Physical Fitness "Convulsive Disorders and Participation in Sports and Physical Education," *Journal of the American Medical Association*, 206 (1968):1291.

should be encouraged to participate in appropriate activities. Such participation should include any sports of interest with the exception of boxing, tackle football, ice hockey, diving, soccer, rugby, lacrosse, and other activities where chronic recurrent head trauma may occur.

Committee reports on just about any subject, not just medicine, do not make easy reading material for most of us common mortals. If both of these reports are read carefully, it is clear that there are two outstanding differences between them. The first report implies that there should be no differences in terms of competitive athletics as long as a child's seizures are under control. The second report does not; it excludes dogmatically all children with a history of seizures from participating in any kind of body contact sports or "other activities where recurrent head trauma may occur." The first report, on the other hand, states that "evidence is meager that closed head injuries [hard bumps] resulting from body contact sports aggravate a preexisting epileptic disorder." We couldn't agree more with this latter statement and the recommendations of the first report. Thus far no proof has been presented to support the belief that recurrent head trauma of the type usually incurred in competitive athletics is a cause of recurrence of pre-existing epileptic seizures. It is the experience of specialists in epilepsy as well as adult and child neurologists, all of whom have had under their care thousands of children and adolescent epileptics who have participated regularly in body contact sports such as tackle football or wrestling, that head trauma sustained during participation in these sports is not a cause of seizure recurrence.

At the time of this writing the American Medical Association Committee on Medical Aspects of Sports is preparing the final draft of a new report which will probably liberalize its 1968 position concerning participation in contact sports by individuals with a history of seizures. Preliminary unofficial reports indicate that the substance of their new position will be along these lines: "Everything being equal, it is probably better to encourage a young boy or girl to participate in noncontact sports. However, if a particular patient has a great desire to play a contact sport and this is deemed a major ameliorating factor in his/her adjustment to school, associates, and the seizure disorder, then serious consideration should be given to letting him/her participate if the seizures are controlled"; and "each patient should be judged on an individual basis."*

An official change on the part of the American Medical Association regarding participation in body contact sports by epileptics—especially football—would certainly give physicians the necessary confidence to allow many of their patients to participate in sports, and avoid in many cases making social outcasts and emotionally crippled individuals of some of these young people, for fear that they may be sued for malpractice should one of their patients suffer physical injury during participation in body contact sports.

Regrettably, the report of the second committee also includes boxing as a body contact sport. It is difficult, if not impossible, for me to place boxing in the same category as football or wrestling. It appears that there are two primary objectives in competitive boxing. The first one is to avoid being hit in the head and the second is to render the opponent unconscious by hitting him in the same place. Just in case you don't remember what you learned in biology class, a K.O. is nothing other than a brain concussion. I believe strongly, therefore, that a "sport" which has as its basic aim the deliberate infliction of repeated brain concussions should be regarded as an inhuman activity and one from which everyone, not only the epileptic child, should abstain.

* *Medical World News* 15 (1974):62B. Reprinted with the permission of the American Medical Association.

Should people then disregard altogether the art of self-defense?

The only skillful and efficient way of becoming proficient in self-defense is by keeping in good physical shape and by learning something like karate or wrestling. Boxing won't get you anywhere except to the floor!

Can a child with epilepsy attend a regular class in a regular school?

We have mentioned several times that a child with epilepsy should lead as normal a life as possible. This general rule applies not only to his everyday activities inside and outside his home but most importantly to his education. If a child with epilepsy is of average intelligence, there is no valid reason why he should not be able to attend a regular class in a regular school.

Some children with epilepsy are intellectually handicapped and will need to be enrolled in special-education classes. It should be pointed out that the need for a particular type of schooling depends primarily on the child's abilities, and not on the fact that he has seizures.

Some children with epilepsy who are of average intellectual capacity may have to attend a special class as long as their seizures are frequent and difficult to control. These include primarily those who experience several grand mal or psychomotor seizures per week or many minor motor seizures per day. Small classes for the instruction of these children are available in many large communities.

Other children with epilepsy may have additional medical problems such as cerebral palsy, mental retardation, or some type of specific learning disability. In these cases, the child may have to be enrolled in a special-education class, in a class for the physically handicapped, or in a class for children with learning disabilities. In spite of average or above-average intelligence, children with learning disabilities may have visual-motor or perceptional or other problems which can make it extremely difficult for them to acquire new knowledge with the teaching methods used in a regular class.

Will seizures affect a child's ability to learn?

Before attempting to answer this question we have to make certain what is really meant by it. This question can be interpreted in two very different ways: first, will recurrent seizures produce changes in the child's brain which will affect his capacity to learn? And, second, will seizures interfere with his ability to carry on his normal school activities? If it were not for the fact that there is always an exception to every rule the answer to the first question would be a resounding "no." In the great majority of children with epilepsy, seizures *per se* do not produce damage to those brain areas responsible for a child's ability to increase his knowledge. Probably the only exception to this rule is the rare occurrence of status epilepticus, which in a few instances may produce irreversible brain damage.

In regard to the second interpretation of this question, there is little doubt that sometimes seizures may seriously interfere with a child's capacity to function properly in school. For one thing, because of very frequent attacks, an epileptic child may miss a large number of school days. Similarly, and this applies especially to patients with petit mal, a child, although physically present, may be missing a great deal of what is going on in the classroom on account of his frequent lapses of consciousness. He may appear to be daydreaming when actually he is having one hundred or two hundred petit mal seizures per day.

Since seizures can be adequately controlled with anticonvulsant medications in approximately 70 percent of children, we can easily appreciate how important it is that a child with seizures be treated as soon as a diagnosis is made, that he take his medication on a daily basis, and that he take it for a prolonged period of time.

What can be done about schooling if a child has very frequent seizures?

Physicians who see a large number of children with epilepsy are frequently confronted with this problem. The child who has frequent seizures needs an education as much as anybody else. He represents, however, a special problem in terms of both treatment and education. Frequent seizures (daily or weekly) may interfere not only with the child's education but also with that of his classmates. This particular situation can best be handled by enrolling the child in a home-bound teaching program. This policy serves the dual purpose of keeping up with the child's education and affords an opportunity for close parental observation during a time when some changes in treatment will have to be made. While the child remains at home, the physician can take the necessary steps to bring his seizures under control. In our experience, a child who has very frequent seizures, other than grand mal, is usually better off at home than in a hospital. Time and again we see children who have several myoclonic or akinetic seizures per day while at home and only an occasional one when they are hospitalized. The explanation of this phenomenon is simple. Unless the child has a private-duty nurse around the clock, regular nursing personnel cannot possibly keep track of all the seizures he may be having during a twenty-four-hour period.

Once the child is seizure-free or the frequency and severity of his attacks have decreased considerably, he can return to his regular school situation.

Can poor school performance or mental dullness in a child of average intelligence be caused by anticonvulsant medications?

Yes, occasionally this can happen. Some children may experience temporary mental dullness as the result of transient elevations in the concentration of anticonvulsants in the blood. This may occur, for example, as a result of a moderately severe infection, dehydration due to various causes, or other situations.

Persistent mental dullness may develop in an epileptic child who was of average intelligence prior to the beginning of treatment with anticonvulsants. If this is the case, consult your physician. Drowsiness, somnolence, and motor and mental slowness can occur if the child is taking an excessive amount of medication or if his body is not able to metabolize and get rid of an amount of anticonvulsant which for another child would be an average dose. In some instances, what appears to be temporary or sometimes prolonged mental dullness may actually be a psychological or emotional problem. It is well known that certain children, especially those with psychomotor seizures, are more prone to develop emotional problems than other children. Many of them are moody, are subject to prolonged periods of depression, have aggressive or hostile personalities, defy authority, refuse to attend school, and sometimes, get into trouble with the law. In situations like these, the physician may have to enlist the assistance of professionals from a child guidance center or refer the child to a psychologist or a psychiatrist.

What can be done if a child with epilepsy is of average intelligence but is hyperactive?

Irrespective of their intellectual endowment some children with epilepsy may also display an unusual degree of hyperactivity (hyperkinetic syndrome). If this is the case with your child, consult your pediatrician. He can evaluate the child's behavior, sometimes in the short interval of an office visit, and decide whether he is a good candidate for treatment with a tranquilizer or a central-nervous-system-stimulant drug. A significant number of these children will improve considerably when given medicines to counteract hyperactivity. In other cases of *apparent* hyperactivity the situation may be much more complex, and in order to get to the bottom of the behavior problem, it may be necessary to enlist the cooperation of a number of people, including parents, teachers, social workers, and psychologists.

What is the hyperkinetic syndrome?

The word "hyperkinetic" means, literally, an excessive amount of activity or motion. "Hyperkinetic syndrome" is the name given to a condition characterized by a marked increase in purposeless physical activity, a short attention span, easy distractibility, and, sometimes, nonintentional destructive behavior. It is not difficult to see how a child with these characteristics may represent a serious problem for parents as well as teachers. It should be emphasized that the hyperkinetic child cannot help being hyperactive. He has absolutely no control over his excessive physical drive. In his mind ideas and interests change continuously from one moment to the other and consequently he is unable to focus his attention on a particular object or situation for more than a very short period of time.

Very little is known about the probable causes of the hyperkinetic syndrome. A number of psychological, social, and environmental influences have been invoked as possible causative or aggravating factors. It is more than likely that biological events taking place during pregnancy or at the time of birth may be important causes of this syndrome. The magnitude of the problem should be emphasized. It has been estimated that approximately five out of one hundred children of school age who are of average intelligence suffer from varying degrees of hyperactivity. For unknown reasons males are affected more frequently than females.

In general, hyperactive children are of normal or above-average intelligence. A significant number of them, however, have specific reading or other forms of learning disabilities. As the child gets older his symptoms decrease in severity, slowly but steadily. Too slowly, perhaps, for parents who can have no rest or are unable to lead a normal family life as long as the child is up and around.

From the child's standpoint, the years from five to twelve are crucial for his educational and emotional development. Thus every effort should be made to carry on a complete evaluation of the child, of his family situation, his school difficulties, his strong and weak psychological areas, and then make the appropriate recommendations for family counseling regarding the child's management, and, in almost all cases of moderate or severe hyperactivity, for a trial of treatment with medications. In spite of average or superior intellectual capacity and marked improvement of hyperactivity with treatment, many of these children may need to be enrolled in special classes for children with learning disabilities.

Are drugs effective in the treatment of hyperactive children?

Yes. Central-nervous-system-stimulant drugs such as Dexedrine or Ritalin have been used for more than twenty years and have been found to be effective in about one-half to two-thirds of children in whom hyperactivity is due to an organic and not to a psychological cause. A lower degree of success is, of course, to be expected when nervous-system stimulants are prescribed indiscriminately to children with all kinds of behavior problems. If a child is going to respond favorably to a stimulant drug, he will almost always do so in a matter of a few days or one week after the beginning of therapy.

How do the remaining one-third or one-half of children with hyperactivity respond to this type of treatment?

When a stimulant drug is prescribed to a hyperactive child one of three reactions can be expected: his behavior may improve, it may worsen, or it may remain unchanged. Since there is no way to predict which child will respond favorably to the administration of stimulants, we have made it a custom to give parents two prescriptions, one for five or six days and another one for two or three months. If the child's hyperactivity worsens, we simply tell the parents to stop the medication; if the hyperactivity improves, they can fill the second prescription. The rationale behind this policy is nothing other than to save the parents a few dollars in case the medication doesn't work.

Central-nervous-system stimulants used in the treatment of hyperactive children can cause insomnia. Because of this undesirable side effect, it is recommended that the medicine be given at breakfast time and, if a second daily dose is necessary, at noon or not later than in the early afternoon. A common complaint from parents of hyperactive children is that they cannot get the child to bed before 10 or 11 P.M. and that, on top of this, he may wake up at 3 or 4 A.M. and just wander around the house. If the child is a natural insomniac, it is obvious then that this problem can only be made worse if the medication for hyperactivity is given late in the afternoon or in the evening.

How can these drugs calm down a child who is hyperactive when they are central-nervous-system stimulants?

The exact mechanism of action of central-nervous-system-stimulant drugs on hyperactive children is unknown. It would seem, however, that their favorable effects are not due to a pep-up action, or to overstimulation, or to a feeling of elation, but to an increase in the child's sensory awareness of his environment. It is quite possible that by increasing sensory awareness, or, in other words, by making the child able to perceive things better these drugs are also able to decrease his motor output and consequently eliminate to a great extent the constant need to touch and explore things and people in order to become aware of their presence. The result is that the child will have a longer attention span and also more organized and purposeful body movements that get him into contact with his environment.

For how long are these children usually treated?

We mentioned above that hyperactivity improves slowly but steadily with advancing age. Unless the child also has severe mental retardation, treatment is rarely necessary beyond the age of eleven or twelve years.

Can stimulant drugs interfere with the action of anticonvulsants in the treatment of seizures?

No. Actually some of these compounds, such as Dexedrine, also have mild anticonvulsant properties.

Are central-nervous-system stimulants toxic or habit-forming drugs?

No. At least not when used when indicated and under a physician's supervision. Stimulants have been used for more than twenty years in the treatment of hyperactive children with no significant toxic effects. If any undesirable side effects should develop, the physician's cessation of therapy or adjustment of dosage will in all instances eliminate any untoward effects or toxic reactions. Drug dependency or addiction has not been a problem in millions of children who have been treated for several years with this type of medication. The situation is comparable to that of millions of epileptic children who have taken phenobarbital or other "potentially habit-forming drugs" for a number of years and in whom drug addiction has not occurred. An entirely different situation, however, exists when these drugs are used in high dosages by emotionally disturbed adolescents or adults. In this regard we should remember that there is a big difference between the use and the abuse of drugs.

In summary, in spite of recent accusations on the part of a few publicity-seeking politicians and a handful of poorly informed professionals that thousands of our schoolchildren are being doped with stimulant drugs, years of experience have proved that there is a definite place for them in the treatment of a large number of children with the hyperkinetic syndrome. We mentioned previously that a diagnosis of hyperkinesis is sometimes easy to make. In many instances, however, this is not the case. It goes without saying, then, that any child with suspected hyperkinesis should be evaluated by a trained physician. Only he can decide whether the child is a suitable candidate for drug therapy or whether he will need additional investigation. Although this kind of therapy is often extremely helpful in decreasing the severity of what is only a symptom, drugs are not curative, and in most cases they are not the only answer to the problem.

What about tranquilizers? Can they be of any benefit to a hyperactive child?

Yes. Until 1954, the year in which a drug called meprobamate was synthesized, there was no truly effective drug for the treatment of anxiety or "nervousness." Up to that time, most of the drugs used in the treatment of "nervousness" or of excessive motor activity also had a significant hypnotic or sedative effect which frequently interfered with a person's activities. Since the introduction of meprobamate, a number of other drugs with the same properties have been synthesized. For the past twenty years, three or four of these drugs have been used with varying degrees of success in the treatment of a large number of hyperactive children. The experience of the past twenty years has clearly demonstrated that tranquilizers are less effective than central-nervous-system stimulants in the control of the abnormal behavior seen in children with the "hyperkinetic syndrome." Nevertheless, the efficacy of these drugs should not be underestimated; there are many instances where they will be effective when central-nervous-system stimulants have failed.

Among the most commonly used tranquilizing drugs are Mellaril, Librium, Chlorpromazine, and Valium.

12. Behavioral and Psychological Problems in Children with Epilepsy

---

Do children with epilepsy experience emotional problems more often than other children?

Yes, they do. And, more often than not, for more than one reason. Emotional problems in epileptic children usually stem from the child's reaction to his condition and from the attitudes of a poorly informed and misunderstanding society. (An exception to this general rule are some children with psychomotor seizures in whom emotional problems are directly related to their seizures and whatever is the cause of them.) It is almost unnecessary to point out in this regard that few if any of us are completely free of emotional difficulties. We all seem to carry into adulthood in some degree, and some more than others, the child within us who needs to be wanted, who desires instant gratification for all his physical and emotional needs, and who longs to be free from responsibilities. A literally translated Spanish adage says: "He who has health, money, and love should thank God for such an abundance of blessings." The epileptic child may wind up having none of these three things, and if the adage were entirely true, he should certainly be among the unhappiest of individuals. He has a chronic disorder with unpredictable manifestations; his road to a successful education and opportunities for employment is often filled with difficulties; and finally, and most importantly, he has to cope with an often misinformed society which still considers him "different" in a very unattractive way. It is ironic that the epileptic, who in the great majority of cases has the capacity to lead a normal life, has to deal not only with a few restrictions and limitations imposed by his condition, but also has to fight prejudices much more frequently than people who suffer from other chronic and much more incapacitating, but for some reason more socially-acceptable, conditions.

Americans so far have failed to develop a sympathetic attitude toward epilepsy and the epileptic. For a long time this country has had popular as well as unpopular diseases. Every year thousands of Americans gladly get rid of millions of dollars, and probably more than a few tears, when famous personalities from the entertainment business remind them in national telethons of the existence of children suffering from truly incapacitating and sometimes incurable conditions such as cerebral palsy or muscular dystrophy. But unfortunately today's list of unpopular diseases is still fairly long, and among them are mental retardation and epilepsy. Thanks in great part to the efforts of a number of national as well as state organizations, however, this list is slowly but steadily growing shorter.

Why do children with psychomotor epilepsy have more emotional problems than children with other types of seizures?

Psychomotor seizures originate in one or both temporal lobes of the brain. The temporal lobes, one on each side of the brain, and structures adjacent to them, constitute what has been called the visceral or "emotional brain." The "emotional brain" determines to a large extent an individual's personality, certain facets of his overall intellectual capacities, such as his ability to memorize recent experiences, and most of his emotional responses.

It has been estimated that approximately 50 percent of

children with psychomotor seizures have some kind of behavior or personality problems. These may become manifested as overt hostility toward peers or relatives, acting-out behavior, aggressiveness, indolence, or outbursts of purposeful destructiveness. Although a young child or a child of school age with psychomotor epilepsy may be unruly or hard to handle and sometimes difficult to live with, he rarely has serious psychologic or psychiatric problems which are so frequently encountered in adults with this type of seizures. In general, behavior or personality problems in children with psychomotor seizures are much more likely to become apparent or to increase in severity at the time of puberty. Also, more serious difficulties are encountered when the onset of seizures is at or after the age of puberty. Psychomotor seizures are relatively uncommon in children under the age of ten; they account for less than 10 percent of all cases of epilepsy in this age period and among such children severe behavior problems are uncommon.

It is important that parents of adolescents with psychomotor seizures and behavior problems realize that these difficulties are part of their child's condition and are not due to something that they have done or failed to do in their relationship with the child. This knowledge can help parents get rid of unjustified feelings of guilt, see their child's problem in an objective way, and consequently be able to face the situation in a more realistic manner.

Is there such a thing as a stereotyped epileptic personality?

No. It was formerly believed that all epileptics were possessed of destructive, egocentric, antisocial, neurotic, and sometimes criminal tendencies. This is sheer nonsense. There is not and there has never been such a thing as a stereotyped epileptic personality. Like any other person each epileptic has his own character and his own unique personality. This misconception regarding the existence of a personality which was common to all epileptics arose originally, and then somehow developed into an accepted "fact," from observations of abnormal behavior in mentally retarded patients who lived in state institutions and who also happened to have seizures. Actually, all that these institutionalized people had in common was the fact that they lived under the same roof.

What can be done if a child with epilepsy also has emotional or behavior problems?

First of all, parents should fully understand that there are no short cuts in the management of emotional disturbances. In the great majority of cases, neither an increase in the dosage of anticonvulsant drug nor a new tablet will do the trick. We have already mentioned that in the great majority of epileptic children emotional difficulties arise not from their condition but from poor adjustment to it and, most importantly, from the attitudes of people close to him. He may be an overprotected child, or he may feel rejected by members of his own family, relatives, teachers, or classmates. All this can certainly make it extremely difficult for him to be able to live like other children.

Where should parents go to get help if they have an epileptic child with emotional problems?

Consult your pediatrician or family physician. Remember, however, that pediatricians and family physicians are extremely busy practitioners. In addition to taking care of hospitalized patients they usually see forty or fifty patients every day in their offices. Everybody should know by now, then, that seldom do they have the time or, often, the interest to take care of children with emotional or behavior problems. Realistic parents shouldn't expect the pediatrician to listen for hours to a discussion of their child's behavior or emotional problems or receive from him a piece of magic "instant" advice for the solution of problems he may not be interested in to begin with. If you believe that your child has a significant emotional problem, simply tell your pediatrician about the problem. If he agrees with you about the nature of it, he will be glad to refer you to a child-guidance center, to a psychologist, or to the appropriate facility in your or a nearby community where your child can get a thorough evaluation and therapy. If you are on your pediatrician's back for too long because your child has behavioral difficulties, the chances that you will get still another prescription to calm down your child's nerves, or that you yourself may wind up taking a tranquilizer, are extremely high.

If the problem is not very serious the child, his parents, or both may benefit from counseling. Most states have child-guidance centers where parents can get the help they need for the common and relatively minor emotional problems seen in childhood. For serious problems, a consultation with a psychiatrist is probably the best thing. Some parents become extremely anxious and occasionally overtly hostile when their physician makes such a suggestion. Since their child is not crazy, why should he be taken to see a psychiatrist? Psychiatry and psychotherapy are helpful in treating a wide range of emotional disturbances and problems, from moderate to severe and stemming from a great variety of causes. Parents ought to remember that the idea that only the insane can benefit from psychiatric therapy is as obsolete as the concept that epilepsy is a disease of divine origin.

How do parents react to having an epileptic child in the family?

In general, in a fairly predictable way. Initially, most parents experience in varying degrees feelings of confusion, anger, or helplessness. For reasons which are difficult to explain many of them cannot help but feel responsible for their child's difficulties. The end result of the parents' inability to overcome these unjustified feelings of guilt can be either overprotection or rejection of the child, especially when seizures are difficult to control, or if, because of heavy financial expenses, other members of the family are deprived of certain amenities. Feelings of guilt often appear to stem from a subconscious suspicion that the child's condition is due to something they did or did not do. The parents of an epileptic child should know that *there is no reason whatever to blame themselves for their child's problem.* The sooner they come to this realization the faster they will be able to rid themselves of feelings of guilt and the better will be the chances of a normal psychological adjustment on the part of the child, and of a more healthy child-parent relationship.

Parental reactions vary somewhat from one family to another. Several factors appear to be of importance in the way parents react to the emotional impact of having a child with epilepsy. To a large extent, factors such as educational background, socioeconomic status and personality and emotional maturity of one or both parents appear to play prominent roles. Unsophisticated parents from low socioeconomic classes and large families are usually little disturbed by having a child with epilepsy. The family has already so many major problems that a child with epilepsy becomes only a mild additional burden. Middle-class parents with strong social and intellectual aspirations appear to be the hardest hit and the least likely to be able to cope with their feelings. Too often many of these parents will manifest a degree of anxiety which is totally out of proportion to the seriousness of the situation. They want and often seem desperately to need an immediate solution to the problem. If for some reason the physician has not been able to win their confidence during the initial visits, it is not unlikely that they will end up in the office of another physician. If they do this, the child may wind up taking two different drugs for several years when probably one would have been sufficient to control his seizures. Worst of all, in some cases they may end up spending hundreds of dollars in the office of a charlatan who has told them that the cause of their child's seizures is a pinched nerve somewhere in the neck or in the back which can be corrected by special exercises or manipulation of the bones of the spine. Parents from high socioeconomic and educational levels are, at least in our experience, the most likely to accept their child's illness and achieve more readily an emotionally stable family environment.

How can parents cope with the problem, relieve their anxiety, and learn to accept their child's illness successfully?

However difficult many parents are to convince about the true nature of their child's problem, the most successful approach appears to depend not so much on a paternal attitude on the part of the physician, but on the time he spends explaining to them a few things that they want to know and a number of others they should know. Parents want to know, for example, what epilepsy really is and what it is not; they want to know why the attacks that a child may have and during which there is no loss of consciousness or jerking of the extremities also have to be called epilepsy. Parents should know at the time of their first visit to a physician that the chances of finding a remediable cause for their child's seizures are extremely low. But also they should know that, even if nothing can be done to eliminate the direct cause of the seizures, there is something that can be done to prevent their recurrence, the type of anticonvulsant medicines available at the present time and their effectiveness, and the chances that the child will "outgrow" his seizures and eventually will be able to get along without medicines. Parents should be told why an epileptic child is supposed to take his medicine every day and for such a prolonged period of time, and also the reason he has to remain seizure free for several years before treatment can be discontinued.

Parents should also know that, if their child is healthy and bright, there is no reason whatever to believe that, because of his seizures or because of the medicines he needs to take, he will lose any of his physical or mental abilities even if he has to take one or more drugs for several years. Many parents are simply appalled when they hear from their physician that, because Johnny had a single grand mal seizure two months ago, he is supposed to take medicines every single day for the next three or more years. Unless they are told that this is the only known way to prevent the recurrence of seizures, the whole thing just doesn't make much sense to them. Parents should understand that anticonvulsant drugs, when taken under medical supervision, will not slow down their child in school and that he will continue to be able to compete academically with his peers; that epilepsy is for all practical purposes not a hereditary condition, and that when he grows up to be an adult he will be able to marry and have children. Parents should also learn that the chances that treatment with anticonvulsant drugs will completely control seizures or appreciably cut down on their frequency are excellent. They should also be aware, however, that in a small percentage of cases seizures just cannot be controlled with any presently available form of treatment.

A clear understanding of the situation can provide more relief than virtually all avenues of emotional support. Parents feel reassured when they realize that their physician knows the problem he is dealing with, and that he will do everything he can to find out the cause of their child's seizures, and that even if this is not possible drug therapy can work miracles. Parents should also know that even if the cause of seizures is

known in the great majority of cases there is very little physicians can do to get rid of it, and consequently the child will
have to receive treatment as if the cause of the seizures was
unknown.

When all the known as well as the unknown aspects about
epilepsy are explained to parents, the greater the chances that
they will be able to accept their child's condition, that they
will fully realize there is nothing shameful about it, that they
do not have to feel guilty about it, and that in the long run
everybody benefits by not hiding the fact that there is an
epileptic child in the family. Parents should also know that it
is far better to have a child with a chronic disorder of the
brain with only intermittent manifestations such as epilepsy
than to have just about any other chronic disease affecting
other organs of the body such as the heart (rheumatic fever),
the pancreas (diabetes), the muscles (muscular dystrophy),
the intestine (cystic fibrosis), the lungs (asthma), or the joints
(rheumatoid arthritis).

How can parents help the child to accept his condition?

It is only when parents have learned to accept the condition themselves that one can expect the child with epilepsy to
be able to accept it in his own mind and at the same time be
able to lead a normal life.

As it was with the parents, the first step in a child's accep-
tance of his disease is a clear understanding of the problem.
The ultimate goal is, of course, to learn to live comfortably
with it and eventually to be able to assume responsibility for
his medications. The child should be encouraged to express
any fears or apprehensions and also be encouraged to ask
questions of the physician during follow-up visits. Children,
even young ones, are smarter and much more perceptive than
most parents realize. Frequently they may not express their
fears or apprehensions verbally, and seem to go around for
months or years as if nothing bothered them when in fact they

are consciously or subconsciously tormented by feelings of insecurity, thoughts of death, feelings of despondency and unworthiness, or downright depression. Let's not fool ourselves about it. The child with epilepsy knows perfectly well that in the mind of many he is considered different from his friends or classmates. And sooner or later he becomes aware that if he happens to have a seizure in school more than one of his peers may make fun of him or make derogatory comments about his condition.

What else can parents do to help the child to accept his disorder and learn to live comfortably with it?

For one thing, they should tell the child about the nature of his problem. This should be done as soon as it is feasible after his first attack or after he has been evaluated by a physician and has begun to take medicines. Any child with epilepsy should know about the nature of his problem at least by the time he enters school. Other children in the family should also be informed of the nature of the attacks their brother or sister suffers. They can then be prepared to answer questions that children in the neighborhood or schoolmates might ask. Parents have to keep in mind that in many cases an epileptic child doesn't know what happens to him during a seizure. He should be told in plain words that he loses consciousness and that often his arms or legs jerk for a few seconds or a few minutes, or that he has short-lasting episodes of staring of which he is not aware, or that sometimes for a period of one to two minutes he loses awareness of what's going on around him and does meaningless things which later on he will be unable to recollect. He should know that this is called "epilepsy" and be told in words that he can understand what the physician has told his parents about the condition. If at all possible parents should avoid being vague and evasive by telling an epileptic child that he has to take a tablet or a capsule three times a day for a couple of years just because the doctor said so. If parents try to hide the facts they are only compounding the problem. They should answer a child's questions truthfully and in words that he can understand. Remember that you as parents have to accept his condition before he does. If parents don't explain to him what epilepsy is and what it is not, somebody else will and that "somebody" may not do a very good job of it. Children are much more cruel and inconsiderate than most people realize.

Unless an epileptic child has very frequent seizures, it is better for parents to avoid starting every other sentence with "You are not supposed to do this or that" and leave it at that without giving him a reasonable explanation. If the physician has told parents that there are certain things an epileptic child is not supposed to do, let him know why. If his ambition in life is to become an astronaut or a professional mountain climber, his parents ought to explain to him that this will not be possible. He may then become interested in something else, develop new interests, turn out to be an avid reader, and eventually be a successful carpenter, lawyer, mechanic, or physician. If the epileptic child knows exactly what's wrong with him, only then can he truly realize that he is not different from anyone else, except that occasionally he may have a brief seizure. He should also understand, clearly, why he has to take medications two or three times daily for such a prolonged period of time. If he knows that their only purpose is to prevent him from having further seizures, he will not feel that this daily ritual is an unjustified ordeal and it will not annoy him as much.

If at all possible, parents should avoid adopting an artificially nonchalant attitude toward the whole affair. No matter how casual they may seem to act, if they still deep down feel that their child is at all times in more or less mortal danger, he will sense the way his parents are reacting to his condition and what they believe are the terrible implications of being an epileptic. Don't let him depend on you for everything. If your child is old enough to understand what happens to him during an attack, do not remind him ten times a day that he has to be careful crossing the streets, walking to the school bus, or going on a bike ride. Moreover, don't be afraid of leaving him alone at home or away from home for a few hours at a birthday party or at summer camp for one or two weeks. Let him handle the responsibilities which every child should be given according to his age and abilities.

It is a well-known fact that seizures may have a profound and long-lasting effect on a child's self-concept and self-esteem. To a large extent, a child's self-concept and self-esteem are determined not only by the awareness he has of his own capabilities but also by the reactions of others around him. If people with whom the epileptic child comes in contact give him a different treatment, either in the form of overprotection or rejection, he is bound to view himself as different and incapable, and subconsciously behave according to the poor image he has of himself.

In summary, if parents fail to accept and, more importantly, to understand his disorder, their child will also fail. The unfortunate result is highly predictable: the epileptic child will live in a state of more or less constant anxiety, in fear of being rebuffed by classmates and friends, and will develop feelings of inferiority, rejection, and isolation, all of which may be manifested as depression or as overt hostile or aggressive behavior. He will fail to develop a mature personality and will end up being an emotionally unstable and unhappy adult, even though his seizures may have been well under control from the very beginning of therapy.

The role played by a child's teacher can be even more important than the role played by the parents. After all, the school-age child spends a great deal more time in direct contact with his teacher than with his parents or relatives—and at an age when he is highly susceptible to the influence of the opinions and reactions of people outside the home. Haven't you already heard, for example, your eight-year-old child telling you how wrong you are about something?—and only because Miss Smith happens to disagree with you! Please do not fail to tell the teacher that your child has epilepsy. If you do not, it is probably because you have not yet fully accepted your child's problem, or because of fear of exposing your child's disorder for social reasons, or for fear that your child might be expelled from school should an attack occur in the classroom. You should realize that, in the long run, hiding and trying to make a secret of the fact that your child is an epileptic can only make things worse both for your child and yourself. A few years ago a survey of approximately one hundred thousand public-school children of Boston showed that in only one hundred and forty-three cases was the teacher aware of having an epileptic child in his classroom. Why didn't teachers know about the other eighteen hundred epileptic children who statistically should have been present in that large number of pupils? I don't need to tell you why. If parents neglect to tell the teacher that the child has had seizures in the past or that he still has an occasional attack, they will probably forget also to inform the supervisor at a summer camp and the parents of children with whom their child might spend many hours away from home. We believe that little is accomplished by this type of policy. We are not recommending that parents discuss the problem with just about anyone with whom their child might come into casual contact. We believe, however, that it is wise that people with whom the child is in frequent contact be aware of the situation.

What about the effect of seizures on other pupils or friends?

Well, there are not too many ways in which one can react. Classmates' or friends' reactions to a child's seizures may be one of fright, or revulsion, or merely surprise. Any lasting psychological effect will depend almost exclusively on the reaction and attitude of the teacher during the episode and, foremost, the manner in which he or she subsequently treats the epileptic child. I said in the previous chapter that should an attack occur in school the teacher can do little to stop it, and that after the attack is over he may end up doing much less of what he can and should do. If the teacher is able to create an atmosphere of easiness and matter-of-factness when an attack occurs in school, he will be able to instill in his pupils a better understanding and a more sympathetic attitude toward the epileptic child. It is also in his power to accomplish much more than that. He can help to reinforce in the mind of the epileptic child the crucial feeling that he is really not different from his classmates.

How should we discipline him?

The child with epilepsy, like any other child, needs to be loved, but he also needs to learn early in life that he cannot always obtain instant gratification for everything he wants. Much too often parents of epileptic children have great difficulties in setting limits on their child's behavior. Parents ought to keep in mind that *consistency* is the fundamental principle on which any type of discipline is based. Parents of children with epilepsy have a strong tendency to become overprotective, to restrict the child's activities well beyond sensible limits, and to be lax about discipline. Overprotection, as well as spoiling, are seldom manifestations of true caring. Moreover, the overprotective parent is also likely to be the one who will end up spoiling the child. Because of totally unjustified feelings of guilt, the overprotective parent ends up giving in to all of the child's desires, no matter how trivial. Let's hasten to add that if parents fall into this trap of indulgence they are probably not giving their child the true love he is entitled to receive, and that if this is the case they too have a real problem, and for their own as well as their child's sake they should seek some kind of help or guidance. Parents don't need to tell a young child that he is loved. He knows better than they whether he is or whether he isn't. And, if a child knows he is truly loved, parents can be absolutely free of fear in crossing him or answering with a firm "no" dozens of his everyday whims. You can be certain that there is nothing else he fears more than losing your love. Sooner or later he will try to please you. The end result of this relationship will be a happy parent and a child who will grow up to be an emotionally mature adult.

Pediatricians as well as other professionals who take care of children never cease to be amazed at the large number of parents who out of the blue appear to realize when their child reaches the age of eight or ten years that he has a mind of "his own." This is, of course, a terrible mistake; for every child has had, since day one, his own and unique mind.

If at all possible parents ought to try to be gentle but at the same time be firm and consistent in their discipline, as they would be with any other child.

Dear parent, be helpful to your child, whether or not he is an epileptic, when he is in some kind of distress. Let him know here and there, by simple body contact—a hug, a kiss, a pat—that you do care about him even if he has done nothing worth a reward. And punish him whenever he has gone beyond the limits you have set for him. A word of caution is in order. If you are able to do it, try to discipline your child without getting very angry. And, if you cannot help getting upset at the time you discipline him, try not to show your anger for more than a moment or two. If you have to punish him in any way, let him know soon afterward that you still love him and act as if nothing of great importance has happened. He will be grateful for the way you react to his mischievous behavior and more than likely will not attempt to repeat it just to get back at you, or try to use his condition to manipulate you or other people around him. Remember that even a young child is able to spot his parents' weaknesses with amazing ease. He may easily find ways to manipulate you, or to use his disorder to make you feel sorry for him, or in a subtle way make you feel guilty for his condition. If you are reasonably confident and strong, and are able to accept and understand your child as he is, you will have no reason to feel guilty. You can be loving and firm. Your child, epileptic or not, will be the better for it.

APPENDIXES

APPENDIX 1. Drugs Used in the Treatment of Seizures in Infancy and Childhood

Drug	Type of Seizure	Preparations	Toxic Effects
Phenobarbital	Grand mal Psychomotor Myoclonic Akinetic Convulsive equivalents	16, 32, 64, and 100-mg. tablets; elixir, 16 mg. per teaspoon	Drowsiness Hyperactivity Skin rashes (rare)
Mebaral	Grand mal Psychomotor	32-, 50-, 100-, and 200-mg. tablets	Same as phenobarbital but occur with less frequency and severity
Mysoline	Grand mal Psychomotor Myoclonic	50- and 250-mg. tablets; suspension, 250 mg. per teaspoon	Drowsiness Unsteady gait Skin rashes Lowering of blood count
Dilantin	Grand mal Psychomotor Convulsive equivalents	30- and 100-mg. capsules; 50-mg. chewable tablets; suspension, 30 and 125 mg. per teaspoon	Gum swelling Unsteadiness of gait Skin rashes Lowering of blood count Excessive growth of body hair Swollen glands
Zarontin	Petit mal	250-mg. capsules; suspension, 250 mg. per teaspoon	Lowering of blood count
Tridione	Petit mal	300-mg. capsules; 150-mg. tablets; solution, 150 mg. per teaspoon	Kidney problems Lowering of blood count Skin rashes
Paradione	Petit mal	150- and 300-mg. capsules; solution, 300 mg. per cc. (1/5 of teaspoon)	Drowsiness Other side effects similar to Tridione (less frequent and less severe)

Drug	Type of seizure	Form	Side effects
Diamox	Petit mal	125- and 250-mg. tablets	Kidney problems Lowering of blood count
Valium	Status epilepticus Myoclonic Akinetic	2, 5, and 10-mg. tablets; ampules for intramuscular or intravenous use	Drowsiness Incoordination (common) Lowering of blood count (rare) Nausea (rare) Skin rash (rare)
Celontin	Petit mal Psychomotor	150- and 300-mg. capsules	Drowsiness (usually transient) Skin rashes Unsteady gait Lowering of blood count (rare)
Milontin	Petit mal	250- and 500-mg. capsules; suspension, 250 mg. per teaspoon	Drowsiness Skin rash Urinary frequency or burning Blood in urine (rare) Lowering of blood count (rare)
Mesantoin	Grand mal Psychomotor	100-mg. tablets	Drowsiness Skin rashes Lowering of blood count
Paraldehyde	Status epilepticus	Ampules for rectal, intra-muscular, or intravenous use	Drowsiness
ACTH	Myoclonic seizures of early infancy	Ampules for intramuscular use	Elevation of blood pressure Intestinal bleeding Increased susceptibility to infections Increase in weight Acne
Prednisone	Myoclonic seizures of early infancy	2.5- and 5-mg. tablets	Same as ACTH

APPENDIX 2. Milestones of Psychomotor Development

Motor	Mental (Social, Language)

One Month

- Infant is able to hold chin up and to rotate head from side to side when lying on his abdomen.
- In all positions extremities are maintained flexed.
- Marked head lag when the infant is pulled by the hands to a sitting position.
- Hands are closed in a fist.

- During first three to four weeks of life, baby has no other way of communicating with his environment than by crying in response to unpleasant experiences (hunger, thirst, pain, etc.). With the exception of the cry associated with colicky pain, all other cries during the first month of life have the same quality.
- By the end of the month, baby learns to regard his mother, and with this he initiates his first meaningful contact with his environment. The ability to regard goes hand in hand with the baby's ability to fix his eyes on people and objects for any prolonged period of time.

Two Months

- When lying on his abdomen, baby is able to lift head to an angle of forty-five degrees from the mattress.
- Less head lag when baby is pulled by hands to sitting position.
- Hands are frequently open.

- Baby begins to smile meaningfully and listen to voices.
- Cry differs according to precipitating factor (hunger, pain, etc.). Mother soon learns to recognize different types of cry.

Three Months

- When lying on his abdomen, baby is able to lift head and chest from mattress, bearing weight on his arms.
- When he is held upright, baby is able to hold head up with minimal wobbling.
- Rolls over from back to abdomen.
- There is lateral arm activity with hands clasped at midline.
- Maintains hands open most of the time.
- Grasps rattle.

- Baby anticipates feeding with increased motor activity.
- Inspects fingers.
- Smiles spontaneously and laughs.
- Begins to babble.

Four Months

- There is no head lag when baby is pulled by hands to sitting, and no wobbling of head when he is held in the upright position.
- Bears some weight on legs.
- Rolls over from abdomen to back.
- Reaches for objects, and begins to appose thumb to other fingers.
- There is finger manipulation of one hand with the other.

- Baby laughs aloud and displays anticipatory response of welcome to mother's presence.
- Baby continues to babble (deaf babies usually stop babbling during this month).

Six Months

- Baby able to sit with support.
- Takes two cubes at a time and transfers a cube from hand to hand. Holds objects with entire palm (immature grasp). Able to reach for objects with one hand several times in a row.

- Strong emotional attachment to mother (or mother figure) already established. Cries if left alone with strangers.
- Babbling continues. Begins to repeat self-made sounds (lallation).

Seven Months

- Sits without support.
- Pulls up to stand from a sitting position if held by hand.
- Holds objects with palm and thumb.
- Tries to get toys which are out of his reach.

- Babbling continues. Says "ma-ma" and "da-da" in a meaningless way.
- Plays peek-a-boo.
- Shy with strangers.

Nine Months

- Begins to crawl.
- Pokes at objects with index finger. Able to hold object between finger and thumb (intermediate grasp).

- Has become increasingly aware and curious about his environment. Seeks attention.
- Anywhere between nine and twelve months, infant begins to recognize words as well as sounds from the environment and responds to a spoken request by perfoming an act such as "bye-bye" or "pat-a-cake." Also begins to imitate gestures and facial expressions, and responds appropriately to his own name.
- Babbling and lallation continue.
- Begins to repeat sounds made by other persons (parrot speech or echolalia).

Ten to Twelve Months

- Walks with assistance or holding on to furniture.
- Begins to walk without help with a broad-based gait by the end of twelfth month.
- Plays with two objects in combination; attempts to take third cube while holding two cubes. Holds objects between tip of thumb and tip of index finger (pincer grasp or mature grasp).
- Interested in pictures in book.
- By the end of the twelfth month is able to understand simple instructions, such as "sit down."
- Says first meaningful word by twelve months.
- Babbling continues.

Fourteen Months

- Walks backward.
- Climbs stairs on all four extremities.
- Able to say three or four single words.
- Responds to simple verbal commands, such as "give me the ball."
- Babbling and echolalia (parrot speech) decrease. At this age exploration of the environment is more important to the child than speech and language.

Eighteen to Twenty Months

- Climbs on furniture.
- Can kick and throw a ball.
- Walks up and down stairs with help.
- Able to build tower of four cubes.
- Feeds self and spills little.
- Vocabulary of about fifteen to twenty-five words, although he is able to understand a much larger number of words.
- Begins to follow directions.
- Begins to use one-word utterances which vary in meaning according to inflection: For example, "Ball?" means "Where is the ball"? and "Ball!" means "Give me the ball."

Two Years

- Can jump in place.
- Can balance himself on one foot momentarily. About 25 percent of children are able to do this by two years; 50 percent will do it by two and one-half years; and 100 percent by three years.
- Builds tower of four or more cubes.
- Helps to undress himself.
- Attempts to fold paper into book form; turns pages in a book singly.
- By the end of the second year vocabulary reaches two hundred or more words and child begins to make two-word sentences. Able to understand a much larger number of words.

Three Years

- Walks downstairs alone.
- Builds tower of nine blocks.
- Unbuttons accessible buttons.
- Able to ride tricycle.
- Can copy a circle.

- Answers in four-word sentences.
- Vocabulary of about nine hundred words.
- Verbal communication is characterized by criticisms, commands, requests, threats, and by questions and answers. Verbalizes toilet needs. Identifies actions in pictures. Names one color. Names most pictures that are commonly found in children's books. Carries on purposeful conversation.

Four Years

- Can copy a square.
- Walks downstairs alternating feet.
- Can hop more than ten steps, and tiptoe ten feet.

- Able to understand between five and six thousand words and to say about two thousand words. Counts to three. Demands reasons ("Why?" and "how?"). Answers in five-word sentences.

Five Years

- May learn to skip.
- Able to balance on toes and to stand for long periods on one foot.
- Can copy a triangle.

- Understands approximately ten thousand words and is able to say about twenty-five hundred words. Answers in six-word sentences.
- Can count to ten and tell his age correctly.
- Reads by way of pictures. Can comprehend story from pictures in book.
- Names the primary colors.
- Can give good definitions for common words in terms of their use.

Six Years

- Learns to tie shoe laces.
- Can ride a bicycle without training wheels.
- Can trace a diamond.

- Vocabulary of about three thousand words.
- Answers in seven-word sentences.
- Able to name penny, nickel, and dime.
- Knows the meaning of morning, afternoon, night, summer and winter.
- Able to relate fanciful tales.
- Recites numbers to thirties.

APPENDIX 3.* **Risk of Epilepsy of Centrencephalic† Origin for Individual with an Affected Sibling or Parent**

	Percentage
Overall basic risk	8
Sibling and one parent affected	13
Sibling affected, both parents unaffected	7
Onset in affected relative before the age of two and one-half years	10
Onset in affected relative after the age of two and one-half years	6
No seizures by age one year	6
No seizures by age six years	2
No seizures by age ten years	<1
Electroencephalogram normal at age five to fifteen years	<1
Affected relative is an identical twin	>80

* Adapted from Julius D. Metrakos, Ph.D., and Katherine Metrakos, M.D.: *Clinical Pediatrics* 5 (1966):540.

† Primary, idiopathic, or metabolic epilepsy.

Index

Acidosis, 122
Acquired epilepsy. *See* Secondary
  epilepsy
Age, epilepsy and, 133–135
Akinetic seizures, 24, 28, 32, 34, 75,
  88, 99, 132, 136, 142, 158, 160, 200
Alcoholic beverages, 176
Alcoholic mothers, 43
American Medical Association
  Committee on the Medical Aspects
  of Sports and the Committee on
  Exercise and Physical Fitness, 195–
  197
Anticonvulsant drugs, 46–47, 49, 83,
  95–121, 143, 169, 199–200, 214–215
  blood levels of, 125–126, 129
  cost of, 130–132
  dosage, 101–102
  effectiveness of, 98–99
  electroencephalogram and, 86–87
  febrile seizures and, 95–97
  history of, 100–101
  mechanisms of action, 97–98
  overdosage, 112–116
  safety of, 103
  side effects of, 109–112, 116–118, 201
  tablets vs. suspensions, 105–108
  withdrawal from, 104–105, 120–121,
    134–136, 170–171
Aortic stenosis, 68

Arteriovenous malformations, 54–55,
  56, 77, 90, 92
Athletics, 174, 193–197
Automatism, 183
Automobile accidents, 50–51
Autosomal dominant, 154
Autosomal recessive, 154
Avery, Roger, 125

Barrow, R. L., 181–183
Battered-child syndrome, 52–53
Bedwetting, 69
Behavioral problems, 201, 208–223
Berger, Hans, 2
Berlioz, Louis Hector, 140
Birth trauma, 39–44, 139, 151, 152
Blood levels of anticonvulsants, 125–
  126, 129
Blood pressure, high, 150
Bonaparte, Napoleon, 140
Brain abscesses, 7, 152
Brain angiogram, 90, 91, 92
Brain damage, 38–39, 45, 52, 57
Brain scanning, 55, 90, 92
Brain tumors, 7, 40, 53, 56, 90–92
Brain-wave test. *See* Electroencephalo-
  gram
Breath-holding spells, 23, 59–64, 166
Bromide salts, 100–101
Bruit, 55

About the Author

Dr. Jorge C. Lagos is a pediatric neurologist at Children's Memorial Hospital in Oklahoma City, Oklahoma, and Associate Professor of Pediatrics and Neurology at the University of Oklahoma School of Medicine. He is a native of Chile, and received his medical education at the University of Concepción and his pediatrics and pediatric neurology training at the Mayo Clinic in Rochester, Minnesota. He has been a resident of the United States since 1961, and was certified by the American Board of Pediatrics in 1969.

Dr. Lagos is the author of numerous scientific papers as well as a medical textbook, *Differential Diagnosis in Pediatric Neurology* (1971). He lives with his wife and two children in Oklahoma City.